Introduction

An autistic child who is able to communicate by computer has written something that looks like this: "I am an Angel descended on Earth for you open the eyes!"

To think of it, it makes you think! The downturn on themselves to these children do it seems not to be the reflection of our own selfishness? The children and the planet we send signs, but we pretend not to see, not to hear them. The only message they send us, it is: "Love Me, help me, take care of me." If the Earth could speak, do tell us it not the same thing?

What is done to these poor little vulnerable beings, thinking of the intoxication due to pollution in all its forms, is strangely similar to what is done to our planet. But because of the parents and physicians have managed to save children of autism, is that it is still time to act. There is always the hope for them, for the Earth and for us!

My son William is a fanatic of Super Heroes. I told him that he is a hero also him since he has saved the lives of several children in the curing of a disease that had hitherto been considered incurable. Later, when it will be great, he wants to become a firefighter in order to be able to save the people. It picks up often debris by land and puts them in the garbage in telling me: "Mom, it is necessary to save the planet!" at school, he received a mention of honor for having cleaned the court. It must know how to read between the lines to understand this message: "The body of children with autism has also greatly need to be cleaned!"

* * *

Before a new ideology to be accepted, it must go through three stages; here is what a proverb says:

1.   "It is first and foremost tour at the ridiculous.
2.   A strong dispute opposes it.
3.   It eventually be accepted as the obvious."

In the history of humanity, how many errors and scientific and medical took place? We only have to think of Galilee. How much time did it taken before that men accept the fact that the Earth is round and not flat and is not the center of the Universe? Galilee was improperly received, it has been tried and sentenced for having dared to tell the truth. Every bearer of the new idea which upsets the ancient beliefs and the pre-set order is perceived as a threat.

When I wrote my first book, autism is not irreversible: how my son has been cured, and that I have presented to my first editor, my manuscript included many more pages. It had proposed to me to publish only the part "testimony" in a first time, in order to leave me time to strengthen the second part by tracing all references of my research. By retrieving the sources of the information already found, and for which I have tried to remain the most faithful possible, I fell by chance on other information just as relevant to complement the first. Therefore, consider this book as the second part of my first book.

Since my first book has sown the controversy, I felt the need to justify myself and explain to the people that I have done so that they can better understand and less judge. I wanted to first and foremost inform my readers on the Biochemical treatment of autism (diet, detox, supplements, oxygen therapy...), but I am told that it would be better to know where comes the enemy in order to better combat.

In the meantime perhaps a next book, I offer you the chance to better understand autism as well as the source of evil in order to know what he will have to work.

Chapter 1

The hereditary factors, the predisposition and the genetic modification

The genetic disorders are not hereditary necessarily

When we speak of the inheritance, it is for the transmission of the characteristics and genetic and biological from one generation to the other comprising the physical and psychological traits. Our body is made up of cells including chromosomes on which are willing of genes with different functions. A dominant gene prevents a recessive gene to impose. However, a recessive gene has need of another recessive gene carrier of the same characteristic appear to see this trait. When a normal gene dominates a abnormal gene, the parent is not reached a hereditary disease; it becomes the bearer of the recessive gene and can pass it on to his descendants. That is why certain hereditary diseases seem to skip a generation. Small changes can therefore occur from one generation to the other until a problem will surface. When the embryo receives its genetic baggage, it cannot escape the abnormal gene from both parents.

The theory based on the heredity as the main cause of autism would have fallen to the water by lack of irrefutable evidence. Despite millions of dollars invested in research , no valid study would not have been able to demonstrate with certainty the existence of a link between autism and heredity. It would have been more promising to guide research on the interactions between genes and the environment.

There is no screening test as is the case for the trisomy during the amniocentesis. A child can be reached of autism without no family history, since any gene could not be identified as the sole responsible.

If the causes were purely genetic, all children within the same family in would be achieved, and at the same level. There is a reason also to which of the identical twins are not met to the same degree. The sharing of a same Environment pre and postnatal would explain autism between members of the same family.

A disturbance in the DNA

Through the evolution, human beings have undergone genetic changes in order to be able to adapt to their new environment and thus be able to survive. The variation of the DNA is therefore due to genetic and environmental factors. For millions of years, new features of character are emerged. During this transformation, external factors have acted on the vulnerability of certain genes at risk, forcing them to wake up, to express themselves or to change.

Parents can transmit to their offspring of genes disrupted. This are the following generations who will be the most affected. Aware of the next few years, if this is not already the case, the percentage of children with autism will be increased by taking unexpected proportions at the point to consider the phenomenon as one of the biggest global epidemics of all time. In effect, the rate of autism would have increased by 300% during the last 10 years. Here is what I heard at a conference on autism given by a physician of the Dan: "A pandemic cannot be caused by a factor purely genetic, and especially not in as short a period of time." (Autism One 2010). So, genetics may not be the only responsible for the emergence and spread of autism.

The human being could well be in the process to go through a period of genetic changes (mutations), because it must adapt to different sources of pollution and changes in their eating habits. Some plant and animal species have disappeared from the surface of the earth or are threatened with extinction because they have not been able to adapt to environmental changes, that they are climate or intakes. Is that what this genetic mutation would put us on the list of the next endangered species if we cannot adapt to it properly?

The change in the genetic material of an organism can create new species. Some of these variations would differ according to the geographical criteria. Sometimes, the consequences can be beneficial or disastrous in the history of evolution. Doctors would believe firmly that autism would simply be a new human race.

The genetic information contained in our DNA plays an essential role in the functioning of our body, and this, on several plans. Some changes in the structure of the chromosomes would affect the normal development of certain cells causing disturbance in the body. The alteration of a cell can cause irreversible modifications of the information that flows between them. The change of the structure of a gene may produce anomalies that can cause a malfunction of the different systems: nervous, digestive, immune, reproductive, respiratory, lymphatic blood,...

The environmental impacts

Environmental factors play a decisive role in the genetic modification. The alteration of the chromosomes would result from exposure to an element external trigger. A bad meeting would alter the function of certain genes among the more likely. The Fragility of a gene would make it more vulnerable to aggression from early from the outside. Regarding autism, it would therefore be of a genetic predisposition. For example, a mutation of a gene could increase the risk that a person suffers from allergies, but to do this, it should be that the latter Between in contact with an agent allergen to trigger a reaction.

Two school buses traveling at the same speed with, on board, the same number of children of the same age. The frontal collision: it is the environmental impact. The shock is almost the same for the whole world. What makes the difference is the place where your child is sitting in the bus. This represents the genetic predisposition. That is why there are who die on the coup; some are disabled for life; others are seriously injured, but with appropriate care, they will succeed to get out with or without sequelae; and some are doing with almost no scratch. (Generation rescue.)

The magnitude of the changes that characterize autism may be explained by the number of genes involved in a form of mutation caused by one or more triggers from the environment. The magnitude and the time of the impact differ in a form of autism another , either innate, is regressive. This is also the reason why there are those who would more easily than others. Everything depends on if the damage is repairable.

The mutagenic agents

The mutated genes or deficient would result of chemical changes in certain parts of the body. The mutation can cause of

4

neuropsychological disorders and disorders of the metabolism. The altered genes may interact among themselves to increase a form of any vulnerability. This sensitivity will therefore be triggered by additional factors such as an aggression from the environment. For example, a child is more inclined to become an alcoholic if its parents were.

The genetic mutations would be more frequent among persons with autism who are beings of more vulnerable and sensitive to chemical pollution. The genetic disturbance in autism would be especially in the gastrointestinal disorders and which would also include a weakness of the immune system. The latter would thus lose its capacity of Well fight the toxins from the environmental pollution. The organization also has a internal pollution. The pollutants involved in chromosomal abnormalities would cause impairment of the immune system, creating a lack of resistance to environmental variation.

The specific circumstances would increase the risk of mutation. All forms of pollution - vaccines, drugs, chemicals, pesticides, heavy metals, genetically modified organisms - can be considered as mutagenic agents. Viral and bacterial infections can disturb the metabolism and create disorder in the biological mechanisms, even going so far as to cause mutations. In some cases, autism may even have been triggered by the intoxication that have suffered the parents; for example, heavy metals may have changed the genetic makeup of sperm and ova. Of chemical substances could therefore interact with DNA. The damage that are caused are derived from attacks from the environment.

Among other agents mutagenic, we would find the electromagnetic waves, the cosmic radiation and X-rays. For example, the ultraviolet rays due to the decrease in the ozone layer could cause errors in the replication of skin cells and cause cancer of the skin. Or, this would be the aluminum and chemical filters contained in the sun creams that would trigger the cancers of the skin. And what could happen in the case of combination of two aggressors?

The body is attacked and he tries to find the mechanisms of defense. Of living beings have difficulty to adapt. Our body is achieved as well as. It even goes so far as to attack its own cells, what is called autoimmune diseases which would part of the autism, the diabetes and, up to a certain point, cancer as it would be in the three cases of a disorder of the immune system. These three diseases would find their origin in an inability to adapt to the modern power supply; that is why a change food may adjust a good part of the problem. The auto-immunity plays a major role since a gene common sensitive link these three diseases. It could prevent the autism in eliminating some environmental factors such triggers that certain foods and chemicals. It would be the same for other chronic and degenerative diseases, also known under the term of diseases of the environment, including a multiple sensitivity to chemicals.

The chemical substances including pesticides, heavy metals and solvents can interact with DNA. The human being as all other species would have difficulty adapting to all these changes. The damage to the DNA would be derived from attacks from the environment and cause changes in the genetic background.

The Triggers

Certain Industrial Chemicals, which are very widespread, contain the incalculable risks, since approximately 80 000 of these substances would never have been the subject of studies prior to their introduction on the market. The assessment of their long-term consequences would never have taken into consideration the high vulnerability of the fetus. A exhibition very early age is more likely to cause long-term problems that exposure to the adult age.

This is not only the dose makes the poison, but also the frequency and the time where the dose is taken. During the first few weeks of pregnancy, pregnant women living near agricultural areas or exposed to pesticides would have more risk of having an autistic child. The intoxication makes the ground more vulnerable, even for generations to come. Even the fact to be exposed to small quantities can lead to defects, mental retardation and autoimmune diseases such as autism. This are the different mixtures of chemical substances that make the cocktail if toxic when a critical step in the development of the fetus.

This are the richest countries and the more industrialized countries who are more prone to cancer, asthma and to autism. The environment interacts with the biological process leading to the appearance of new diseases chronic diseases. Internal and external pollution would therefore on the physical and intellectual development Normal: these harmful particles would create blockages in the gear of different mechanisms.

The diseases associated with an immune dysfunction are in full expansion. The aggressions early environmental trigger these anomalies which disrupt the functioning of the immune system and weaken it. Our defense system can not cope with all these attacks. Prenatal stress, which follows, would cause of tensions mental and

6

physical. Too of adrenaline can decrease the capacity of natural defenses. We catch often a cold after having lived strong emotions; it is a little bit the same here. An increase in the stress hormones can change the fetal development. We still do not know all the biological effects on health and the consequences on the pregnancy. The stress, including the oxidative stress, could therefore have an impact on the health or increase the vulnerability to diseases.

The pollution caused by the electromagnetic waves would also play a role in the detoxification process cell. The irradiation of wireless communication devices would cause cracks on rays of DNA. This cell disruption would ensure that the toxins remain imprisoned in the body. The progression of autism would have appeared at the same time that the technological evolution. This would be only a coincidence?

The interactions between the brain and the immune system are to ensure that the brain has its own local responses immunity and inflammatory. If one considers the vaccines as the aggressors of the immune system, it can also be considered as a form of stress as well as a trigger important. Proteins can be produced by the presence of foreign substances toxic and harmful become themselves to the organization. The wounds caused by a lack of oxygen would trigger a process abnormal inflammatory that can lead to neurological disorders. Of the mechanisms of defense inappropriate would contribute to the development of Alzheimer's disease, multiple sclerosis and autism, because an overproduction of antibodies will damage the neurons and would prevent the red blood cells carry oxygen to carry out their work.

It qualifies the diseases of the environment as a multiple sensitivity to chemical products and everything that is not natural. There is therefore a link between the environment and its impact on health.

The genetic mutation spontaneous

The weathering, which is the unusual mutation of a gene or genes, may occur at the time of the fertilisation if there has been contact with a environmental aggression early. Congenital malformations may have been caused by the abuse of drugs, medicines and alcohol. The Fetal Alcohol would trigger a genetic predisposition to autism. The antidepressants would decrease the functions of the immune system impeding the detoxification process, which may have an impact on the development of the fetus. The anticonvulsants taken during pregnancy would also be criminalized. It seems even that the influenza vaccine given to pregnant women would contribute to neurological disorders in the fetus. Other elements irritants can have been introduced before, during or after pregnancy and childbirth as the hormones to increase the contractions and the epidural anesthesia. It is of risk factors which may therefore contribute to the development of autistic disorders since they can be considered as the aggressors.

The expression of a gene is done at a certain time given during development. A gene may not be shown correctly during the training cell. Research have attempted to demonstrate the responsibility of the Y chromosome to explain the highest rate of autism among boys than girls. These have two X chromosomes and when an error occurs on one of them, the other can repair, which is not the case for the XY chromosomes. The incidence of autism in three boys for a girl would find its justification in the genetic factors or hormone levels.

The genetic mutation spontaneous would be the result of an error committed by the cell when it copies the information of its DNA before dividing. It is a mistake that the mechanisms of repair would not have been able to detect during the fertilization or throughout the embryonic development. The system for the repair of DNA, which has the function to correct errors in replication, may have been the subject of a change when a cell division influenced by exposure to a mutagen. A spontaneous mutation genetics would promote the autism. "The same thing happens when we transcribe a text. Although we try not to make many spelling errors, even rereading, we do not always find." (Paris Conference.)

The age of the parents

In our days, the couples choose to have children much later in their life, putting first their priorities on studies and on their career. The important thing is to found a family on solid bases. Studies have tried to blame the age of the father to explain the increase in autism, but if one considers that the target population consisted of the Fathers of more than 30 years, it is not surprising that the data confirmed what they were trying to prove.

Regarding the age of the parents, the only possible avenue to consider would be the following: more one is elderly and more our Organization has had the time to store toxic substances which may have damaged some genes, especially if the parent has often been in contact with chemical products, toxic and hazardous wastes.

Our DNA evolves throughout our lives. The spontaneous mutation would grow with the age, which would make it more likely elderly parents to have children with autism. With age, the repair of DNA would work with less effectiveness. The more it is old, more our cells making mistakes in the retyping.

The vacuum at the Autism

A lot of psychiatric illnesses have been discovered in the families of children with autism. Among these, we would find the depression, personality disorders, epilepsy, schizophrenia...

The genes have been associated with the production of energy for the neurons. A deficit on this plan would create a lack of synchronization in the activities of the brain. A gene altered would therefore have the responsibility to produce a protein facilitating communication between neurons, and other proteins may harm this operation. The transportation of the serotonin is essential to the operation of the neurotransmitters. So there could be a link between autism and mental illness of some parents (for example, if there is one who suffers from depression).

The origin of the psychiatric disorders would be of gastrointestinal disorders. It must be considered that this are the intestines which feed all the organs of the body. The brain can therefore suffer from nutritional deficiencies.

Celiac Disease

Genetically speaking, our Organization would not be made to digest some current food, especially with all the chemicals they contain and which can damage our intestinal mucosa. There are a few billion years, our food was limited to the meat, fruits and vegetables. Thousands of years ago, cereals have emerged and have become our basic food.

The genetic diversity of the species of grasses would have been reduced by the selection of species by the hand of the man and by the Natural selfing of the fields. The intensive production has taken the place of the genetic manipulation natural. Among the mutant species, those who had a better fastening of the seed on their ear and a greater amount of grain would have been selected to the detriment of other species that exhibited a greater ability to clump together. It is as well that would have appeared the gluten in our power.

Through the centuries, some peoples, at different places on the planet, have adapted to new nutritional elements, but they have had much more time for us to do so. So we have not had the time to adapt to changes fast food.

Celiac disease could well find themselves among the diseases of the century. More and more people become intolerant to gluten, and most ignore or refuse to recognize. The lactose intolerance would be caused by the sensitivity to gluten, since the latter, spoiling the intestines, would be responsible for the destruction of enzymes intended for the digestion of dairy proteins. All the people who are lactose intolerant could also have a hidden intolerance to gluten. It is as well as food intolerances can trigger other. The destruction of the enzymes responsible for the degradation of gluten could have been caused by intoxication to heavy metals some of which would come from several vaccines, of certain drugs, as well as by the power supply, some pesticides that contain also the heavy metals.

The toxic nature of intolerance to gluten would have raised a variety of new physical and mental illness: Autism, hyperactivity, epilepsy, schizophrenia, anemia, anxiety, arthritis, cancer, nutrient deficiencies, colitis, constipation, diarrhea, diabetes, depression, learning difficulties, food intolerances including that to lactose, chronic fatigue, fibromyalgia, thyroid disorder, infertility, pancreatic insufficiency and renal, liver disease, Crohn's disease, irritable bowel syndrome, poor functioning of the gallbladder, obesity, disruption of enzyme system, eczema. Signs of this intolerance was would recognize by black rings under the eyes may indicate a bad absorption of iron, without forgetting the fact of having the pale complexion, white spots on the enamel of the teeth and a belly pot-bellied. Physical factors may impede the development and functioning of the brain. In this case, the mental illnesses can be derived from physical diseases. "A healthy mind in a healthy body", as said so well the saying.

Intolerance to gluten destroys the intestinal villi (filaments) which have as a function to draw the nutrients in the feed. In the case of a poor functioning tract and of a defect of the villus, it is certain that the entire body suffers from nutrient deficiencies. For example, if milk products cannot be digested properly, then it is impossible to absorb calcium. If the lymphatic system is poorly fed, he will not be able to function well; The same applies to the other systems and organs, which can lead to chronic diseases, among other diabetes and autism.

Some minerals would be responsible for the intake of oxygen to the cells. This lack would explain the reasons for which the therapy by oxygenation under pressure by hyperbaric chamber seems to be effective for feeding the cells injured by this deficit in oxygen. The oxygen helps the bodies to operate better; it is at the basis of life on Earth. Our brain has need of oxygen, and yet we offer him of the pollution.

The brain lack of essential nutrients to work well, which, in several cases, may have been caused by gastro-intestinal disorders. A bad absorption of food by the intestine damaged creates nutritional deficits. The increase of neurological diseases may therefore have a link with the celiac disease.

Here is a story that I read in a science magazine whose name escapes me:

A woman will see his doctor because she eats a book of small sheets of paper per day. Could not prevent, she believed that she had become mad. The doctor knew that this kind of behavior could be caused by a lack of vitamins or minerals. It is therefore spend taken of blood and realizes that its rate of iron is very low. Then, he prescribed an iron supplement that she takes religiously for several weeks, but this has not solved its problem. He knows that if the iron cannot be absorbed, it is because the intestines function poorly. He is therefore pass other tests and he discovers that she is reached of the celiac disease. It makes him a gluten-free diet. Since then, she has no more never had the taste to eat of the paper.

Some children with autism have a behavior similar to this woman: they lick the walls, furniture or objects to the search for minerals whose body has need, because their system attempts to compensate by its own means. Among the signs of possible anemia are a pale complexion, a lack of energy and a lack of concentration. This are similar symptoms to the intolerance to gluten. Some children with autism are similar to children in the third world: meager, without muscular tone with a swollen belly. The lack of iron is therefore a sign of the celiac disease, since the intestines damaged cannot absorb it. The lack of iron in the blood would also reduce the intake of oxygen to the cells.

The symptoms of a certain form of autism are strangely like those of the celiac disease; that is why several children recover after a diet without gluten or casein which make disappear most of the symptoms associated with autism, as well as to the celiac disease. Intolerance to gluten can therefore be part of a genetic predisposition to autism. In this case, parents with celiac disease could very well have an autistic child.

The radical changes in our food supply, including chemical products that are there, have been able to force our DNA to change in order to be able to attempt to adapt. We only have to consult the lists of ingredients on the packaging of all processed products on grocery store shelves for us to realize that there are of the Wheat (gluten) as well as its other derivatives in almost everything. We do not have the genetic makeup of the Asians to digest well the soybean.

Some new imported foods, which are suddenly arrived in our power, can be considered by our organization as foreign bodies. By a lack of addiction, the immune system would deal as intruders and for the combat, it would produce antibodies to the origin of food allergies.

Chapter 2

The affective disorders

The lack of love

The system conventional medical would have thought for a long time that the family and social environment played a role in the emergence of the autism. It accused the poor mothers of not having given enough attention and given enough of love to their child, what he called "the syndrome of the mother cold". The Psychiatric Institute preached in the 1960s the myth of the mother guilty:

[...] The consequence of the autism was notably due to the parental attitude cold and devoid of affection [...]. It was mainly the character of the mother who was often put in question by its inability to establish a communication with his child. The latter, not finding answers to its need for communication, désinvestissait little by little the outside world and is contained on itself without exchange with the environment. It is a thin up to become a fortress empty.[1]

At the time, the Autism was therefore considered as the result of a lack of affection as a result of an infant psychosis. Separate the baby's mouth too early the nipple of his mother could cause the loss of the sense of existence and of belonging resulting in an agony primitive. It accused the parents to be the cause of the disorder of their child. They were blamed to be little magnets, too intellectuals and rigid.

The cold relations between parents and children were regarded as decisive factors in the development of his personality. The child who felt rejected could not find its own identity nor recognize themselves in the world as part of and as desired person. The inability to establish a communication mother-child came, after the connoisseurs in the matter, a maternal fantasy unconscious of murder.

At the time, treatments consisted to separate the child from his mother in the removing of the family environment. The feeling of guilt was enormous and unbearable for the parents. This thought has hardly changed with time. Programs for the rehabilitation of some centers claim that to treat autism from the child, it is necessary to change the behavior of the parents under the pretext that they do not know how to communicate or how to play with their child. The paternal absenteeism has also been, for a long time, pointed the finger for having participated in the sense of rejection.

The medical opinion has changed little with time. A GP specialist in psychiatry even told me: "What makes children with autism, it is because the mothers do not know how to say "I love you" to their child nor how to show them their love." Today, other theories on the horizon, the excess of which stress, the birth of another child, a recent separation and the postpartum depression. Especially do not believe someone who will tell you: "Your child is autistic become because you do the watched not long enough in the eyes when thou allaitais, that is why his brain has not developed a visual contact."

Even if the maternal presence is very important during the first two years of the life of the child, this does not take away the fact that a mother who does not work and which remains in the Home may very well also have an autistic child. Lay the blame on the backs of the other is an excellent way to déculpabiliser, is it not?

Too of love

Not knowing more too what to say, the Middle pédopsychiatrique would believe firmly that autism is now due to "a too-full of love", and that the mothers are become too dedicated to their child. It passes therefore from one extreme to the other. Seek the black beast where there is not is an excellent way to divert the truth and to flee the reality. That is the real causes and that it condemns the real culprits! Is it that the specialists would be blinded by their lack of knowledge, their recklessness, or would it be that of ignorance, pure and simple?

What would be more likely, and this is only a hypothesis is that a surplus of affection and protection would prevent the child to explore its environment in the search information, what constitutes an important exercise to promote the stimulation of the five senses as well as the physical and intellectual development, especially if the parents have too much of a tendency to take Often the child in their arms. Is that too much of love and attention can be harmful to this point?

A child from a family environment where reigned the violence had of autistic symptoms and those it would have decreased when it has been placed in a host family. Then we must ask if his new environment of life was not simply less polluted. It should also consider the food change. If the changes in the environment can alleviate the symptoms, it should explore more conscientiously the environmental impacts in the triggering of autistic symptoms.

Chapter 3

Pregnancy

My child is with autism by birth, by regression, or a combination of the two?

The presence of environmental factors during pregnancy could trigger a mutation and a genetic predisposition to autism. It seems that the third of children with autism are for the birth. It can therefore be, in some cases, of something innate. However, regarding autism by regression, the symptoms first appear as a result of a particular event that acts as a trigger. The environmental impact may take place before, during or after birth. The intoxication of the child can therefore begin inside the belly of the mother and continue thereafter.

Malnutrition

The supply of the pregnant woman is very important because it is this which nourishes the fetus which must not be missed of essential nutrients in order to ensure its normal development.

An unhealthy nutrition would be due in part to a form of poverty. The financial concerns of families in debt in the most industrialized countries as well as the mode of modern life (fast food and prepared meals) would play a role regarding the nutritional deficits. A bad absorption in the mother would deprive the fetus of essential elements.

A intoxication on several plans

In principle, the food should not contain toxic products that could harm our health (flavor enhancer, flavors and artificial dyes). However, recent studies in the United States would have demonstrated that the contact with chemical and hazardous products such as pesticides, PCBS, solvents and dioxin during the period of gestation could compromise the development of the brain of the fetus and thus disrupt the functions of the nervous system. For that the baby develops normally, it is still necessary that the mother be immune to the toxic products.

The period, the duration, intensity and the proximity of the exhibition are fundamental elements. Pregnant women or in Age of the become should refrain from work in places where they are in contact with dangerous products. I have known of the mothers of children with autism who have worked in greenhouses, hair salons or with products of housekeeping powerful. Women of childbearing age, living on farms or near agricultural areas would have more risk of having an autistic child.

The exposure to organochlorine pesticides would disrupt the development of the nervous system of the fetus. The first eight weeks of pregnancy are more crucial and decisive and vulnerable. The brain of the fetus is extremely sensitive and fragile at this stage of its development. Autopsies have shown the brain lesions that were held in the first quarter of the pregnancy. In some cases, the neurological damage is irreparable.

Even if we had been led to believe for a long time that the placental barrier and not brain let pass only a tiny part of residues, analyzes would have demonstrated the presence of traces of pesticides, PCBS, of release coatings, of dioxin and other toxic substances in the blood content in the umbilical cord. This would be the reason for which all the umbilical cord are sent to the laboratory for analyzes which it does not intend to speak. Traces of pesticides would have also been found in analyzes of urine of pregnant women. In addition, some herbicides and insecticides would trigger of the anomalies in the development of the immune system.

"The mothers who used shampoos to basis of pesticides for Washing animals (domestic) while they were pregnant had a risk two times larger than their child suffers from a autism spectrum disorder."[2] The polluting products used in the renovations and the construction of new housing such as varnishes, paints, glues and solvents would explain the increase in cases of autism in the rich countries. I was surprised to find, in doing my consultations in the home, the number of children with autism living in these beautiful large mansions new which resemble castles. The exposure of a pregnant woman to solvents would multiply the risk of malformations.

The products of housekeeping can cause a delay in the maturation of the immune system. The perfumes would disrupt the hormonal mechanisms of the fetus. The plastics containing bisphenol with which the bottles were manufactured during long are toxic when they are heated. It took several years before the government on the Prohibition of the use in the manufacture of plastic containers. He must believe that the population served as a guinea pig to test products. Why not have tested its toxicity before its implementation in market?

Millions of people would be achieved, without the knowledge, environmental hypersensitivity to chemicals which are also multiple that PCBS, dioxins, fungicides... The exposure to even low doses to these neurotoxins would also play a role in the increase of the hyperactivity, attention deficit, the difficulties of learning and conduct disorders, all cousins of the great family of the autism.

Pre- or postnatal exposure to relatively low concentrations of three substances in particular, namely the lead, PCBS and methylmercury, has been associated with a slight decrease of neurological function and intellectual [...]. The exposure to certain toxic substances including lead, manganese, solvents, dioxins, PCBS and pesticides has been to various degrees in link with attention deficit disorder with hyperactivity.[3]

The chemicals would therefore also responsible for intellectual disabilities including a decline in the average of the IQ (intelligence quotient). Millions of deaths each year would be allocated to pesticides and the pollution of the atmosphere. Exposure to household cleaning products or industrialists and punishment as well as the cosmetics, lead, mercury, PCBS during pregnancy may lead to a brain dysfunction in the child as well as a decrease in the size of the cerebellum. The maquillants products, which contain lead and mercury, can penetrate in our system by being absorbed by the skin.

The PCBS would be part of the most toxic substances, the more persistent and more polluting. They would decades before disappearing completely from the environment. Even if their use is prohibited for years, these substances remain in the air, water and soil. In occurring on plants and in the flesh of the animals that we eat, it is as well that they go to the food chain up to the human being. Our food would therefore be contaminated. Being hyposolubles, dioxins thus remain in the fat bodies whose meat, milk and eggs, and then the bone marrow and the brain.

The dioxin would be part of endocrine systems immune, nervous and reproductive. It would also be highly carcinogenic. If it has indeed a impact on the DNA, it could also cause a genetic mutation.

He must believe that the government would have lost the control of industrialization, agriculture and the agri -food industry with the multinationals, or he would have been influenced by the lobbying.

Alcohol and Tobacco

The consumption of alcohol and tobacco can affect the development of the fetus. Certain drugs and narcotic drugs increase the risk of foetal malformations. The mother who consumes alcohol during her pregnancy has more at risk of having a child with autism: this is what is called "Fetal alcohol syndrome".

"The alcohol induced the same damage to the brain that rubella."[4] which would mean that the rubella vaccine could cause damage to the brain.

The alcohol acts directly on the development of the brain and the nervous system of the embryo and the fetus, because it can more easily pass through the barrier of the placenta. The liver of the baby does not yet work well enough to be able to eliminate it properly. The results would be among the following: disorders related neurological development, intellectual retardation, a fetal malformation, a premature birth, psychiatric disorders, aggressive behaviors, heart abnormalities, babies of small size. A premature baby has a greater risk of developing the Autism.

"A Swedish study has shown that smoking in early pregnancy increases (to 40% probability) the risk of having a child who suffers from autism."[5] smoking during pregnancy restricts the growth of the fetus. The carbon monoxide would decrease the quantities of oxygen that can create a form of anorexia. It contracted the blood vessels and increase the blood pressure, which would send less oxygen in the blood to cells. A Mortality in utero may then occur. The nicotine would affect the behavior and the mood in the adult. Children exposed to cigarette smoking would therefore be more likely to have antisocial behaviors. If, during the fetal period, exposure to tobacco smoke is permanent, this would increase the risk of having a child with a mental illness or physical. It must not be forgotten that tobacco smoke contains cadmium and arsenic, toxic heavy metals, and that several children with autism are intoxicated by the latter.

Among the child, exposure to cigarette smoke pre and postnatal can also increase the possibility of Be reached a Attention Deficit Disorder with or without hyperactivity or of the underhanded celiac disease. In addition, during pregnancy, tobacco would increase the potential for physical infirmities at the ends of the body. But what is it that can then cause autism in a child whose mother has never taken drugs, nor of drug or alcohol and who did not smoke?

The hormones

If there is a link between the beginning of a pregnancy during that the mother takes again the birth control pill and the lack of what is called "the yellow body" essential during the formation of the embryo at the primary stage, is that the taking of synthetic hormones could have a role to play in the triggering of the autism. How many of the women who took the birth control pill have had a child with autism? A hormonal factor could be one of the causes of autism, since this disease affects more boys than girls.

A high level of testosterone would lead to an increased masculinity of the brain. Too high a rate of the male sexual hormone in the amniotic fluid would expose it the child to a hormonal dysfunction? Or again, the hormones present in the flesh of animals that we consume in Would they be responsible?

The yeasts and Candida

The decision of the birth control pill over a long period would encourage the proliferation of intestinal yeasts thus impeding the functioning of the immune system.

A mother infected by a candidiasis in pregnancy or childbirth can infect the baby. Intestinal parasites such as Candida albicans produce tens of toxins which can affect the neurons. The intestinal yeast can pass through the intestinal mucosa, it itself has damaged, and enter the bloodstream where it does feeds more waste as was the case during his stay in the intestines, but of nutrients essential to its host. The toxic waste products by this parasite cause damage to the body and affect the functioning of the digestive systems, nervous and immune systems. In addition, the porosity of the intestinal wall caused by its passage opens the door to the Food particles (triggers allergies) and to proteins badly digested.

A good part of the useful bacteria in the intestinal flora natural would not have just been destroyed by the pill, but also by the antibiotics, by heavy metals, by chemotherapy, by the surgeries, by a diet rich in starch and sugar, by pollutants, by lack of exercise and oxygen.

The magnetic radiation

It seems that the new light bulbs in spiral (those that contain mercury) emanate from the electromagnetic waves of a great power. And this is not all.

According to the doctor Richard Lathe, batteries of mobile phones abandoned in the nature or buried in landfills would be responsible for the significant increase in cases of autism in the United Kingdom, because of the many heavy metals that they release. The radio waves emitted by these devices affect the blood-brain barrier that separates the blood of the brain and make it more porous. Less waterproof, this protective barrier of our brain leaves penetrate of toxic substances, heavy metals, in particular. As well, for some researchers, the strong and recent increase of autism cases could in part be attributed to the resurgence of electromagnetic radiation emitted by mobile phones. The radiation emitted by these phones would be able to retain the heavy metals in the cells by preventing their elimination. The effect is all the more serious in that these same radio waves emitted by the notebooks interfere with the dental amalgam increasing the release of mercury.[6]

And what can we say about the batteries of the toys from children and of other electrical devices, including appliances?

The ultrasound

Ultrasound examinations performed on animals would have disrupted the development of the brain of the fetus.

"Among the pregnant mouse subjected to Ultrasound, a small number of nerve cells of the cortex of the fetus does not arrive to develop properly in the cerebral cortex."[7] Some brain cells are incorrectly remained dispersed to other locations and have not been able to develop normally or to establish connections between them. The duration of the ultrasound has an impact, but this would depend on the size of the brain and the stage of development of the fetus. That is why it should be avoided to make unnecessary examinations as if it were a pure entertainment, to the detriment of screening of diagnostics justified.

Mercury

The mercury is part of the more toxic chemicals to which the child would be the more exposed before coming to the world. It would affect the neurons by disrupting the biochemistry of the different steps in the development of the brain of the fetus, which is much more sensitive and vulnerable than that of an adult, especially at a critical period. The intoxication may come from the liberation in permanence of dental amalgam of the mother to each chewing.

A study establishes that children with autism have higher rates of mercury in the body as the children not achieved. According to the study, children with autism have also been treated more than the other by antibiotics at the bottom age. The use of antibiotics is known to prevent almost totally the excretion of mercury given the alterations of the intestinal flora that they cause. Thus, a higher use of oral antibiotics in children with autism has been able to reduce their ability to excrete mercury, which could explain the high rates of mercury stored in the body of these children.[8]

The reduced amount of mercury in the hair analysis proves that this heavy metal remains fixed in the organs (including the brain) instead of going out of the body.

The vaccines during pregnancy

The vaccines during pregnancy would be part of the risk factors that contribute both to the development of autism that exposure to paints, tobacco and pesticides. If they are not directly responsible, they are at least of the major triggers of a functional imbalance leading to anomalies. A high percentage of mothers with a child with autism have a blood type Rhesus negative.

The injections of immunoglobulin to all pregnant women with an HR-, regardless of the blood type of the biological father, would have coincided with the significant increase in autistic disorders in recent years, but the medical authorities still say that it is only a coincidence. The high use of the Rhogam would expose the mothers to repeated doses of mercury during a critical period of the development of the fetus, which could impede its neurological development. The study which claimed the contrary would have been financed by the manufacturer of the vaccine itself.

What can we say about the vaccines against the flu that receive the pregnant women and which contain thimerosal? When a doctor said to a mother: "the flu vaccine will protect your baby", should it not say to the place: "This vaccine contains mercury and a virus that can intoxicate your baby and make it seriously ill"? Or again, instead of asking us if we are allergic to eggs before inoculation, should it not rather ask us if we wish to become intolerant to eggs and poultry? Because this is not normal to receive of animal proteins through the skin instead of digestive tract without reacting the immune system.

The virus during pregnancy

The brain lesions in the brain of the baby may have been caused by a viral infection during pregnancy. Microbes such as Streptococci and syphilis can lead to psychiatric disorders. If syphilis can make people crazy, what is the potential of other viruses including those who are injected? Approximately 20% of mental illnesses would be due to prenatal infections such as that of the flu. The flu vaccine can therefore cause the same damage as the flu itself.

The disease the most obvious is the schizophrenia, but autism, bipolarity (manic depression) and Disorders Obsessive The behavior could be related to viral infections, bacterial or parasites in utero, during the early childhood or of the childhood [...]. Some of these infections directly affect the brain, but others generate a reaction of the body which makes interference in the development of the brain and even which attacks the cells of the brain by error auto-immune.[9]

If the mental illnesses can be caused by microbes, then we must ask questions about the vaccines administered to women before, during and after the design, as well as those given to infants, children, adolescents, adults and the elderly; without forgetting the phenomenal amount of prescribed medications (antihyperactivité, antidepressants, antipsychotics, etc.) which must bring in a lot of money to the pharmaceutical companies.

Mental illnesses would be attributable to a disorder of the immune system. Abnormalities of the immune system triggered by attacks early environmental would be responsible for chronic diseases and neurodevelopmental disorders. The pandas (Pediatric Autoimmune neuropsychiatric disorders associated with Steptococcal Infection) develops from the immune system that attack the brain after the infection. Streptococcus produces a protein similar to another; that is why the immune system attacks its own cells of the body. The development of the brain is interrupted by this auto-immune response. Children who have been affected by a streptococcus have developed by the result of the neurotic condition the behavior (TOC).

The parasites and the toxins that they emit can transform the personality of their host in affecting the chemicals in the brain, which damages the development and the operation of the latter and changes at the same time the emotions and the behavior of the person. Psychiatric illnesses can therefore be caused by influenza, by the rubella and by the herpes. The MMR vaccine contains the living virus of rubella. Experiments conducted on mice have revealed a lack of curiosity and social contacts as well as a fearful attitude as a result of these inoculations. An autopsy showed differences in the distribution of neurons. The MMR vaccine can therefore cause the same damage to children and to pregnant women whose their fetus.

A high percentage of women who have received a live virus vaccine for rubella before the design would have had a child with autism. If the mother suffers from immune diseases, the risks are greatest; without forgetting the number of miscarriages possible, of mortalities Natales and sudden deaths of the infant. It is not yet known if it is of the infection itself or of the response of the immune system, or even of the antibodies produced against these microbes which would cause the damage.

The herpes virus can go to the fetus during pregnancy. Some people are carriers without symptoms. The barriers of the placenta and encéphaliques would not be as leakproof as it might seem. The immune defenses weakened by the mother or the immaturity of those of the fetus would not fight effectively against the virus.

Better diagnostics do not explain the increase of autism. In addition, an epidemic is not caused by genetic factors, but rather by viruses and by bacteria, which may include those who we are injected. Inject viruses would be like shooting itself in the foot. Is this a form of autism would be due to an autoimmune attack caused by the virus, by bacteria, parasites and other microbes that will destabilize our immune system? In addition, all of these microbes can produce toxic proteins; therefore, it could be a form of poisoning.

The predisposition to autism would thus include immune disorders. And who are responsible?

The antibodies

Among the mothers who have received the vaccine measles, mumps, rubella (MMR) before the design, 78% of them would have had a child in the autism spectrum. In addition, the living virus passes through the breast milk and may thus continue to affect the child.

"The women who are not able to produce protective antibodies after having received live vaccines pose a immune dysfunction that predisposes to have children with autism."[10] Too antibodies in the blood can block the more small blood vessels depriving the cells of oxygen and nutrients, or attach to the cells of the brain and the damage. Even the opiate proteins of a mother suffering of intolerance to gluten and casein could cause the same damage to the fetus, to his brain and to his intestines.

The Immune System

The diseases associated with immune dysfunction would be on the rise. The brain possesses its own immune defenses which are sometimes produced by a substance created by the immune system main. Inflammation of the brain may result.

Of attacks suffered by the immune system in full development of the fetus or the child may lead to a consistent pattern of effects that can induce different diseases in adulthood. Among these pathologies, discusses the neurological disorders, allergies and the anomalies autoimmune diseases, the deletion of the response to vaccines, as well as an increased risk to infections, cancer and a number of other chronic diseases.[11]

Exposure to the following elements are risk factors likely to disrupt the early development of the immune system: PCBS, herbicides, pesticides, heavy metals, fumes of oil and diesel. The consumption of alcohol and tobacco as well as the use of hormones and antibiotics in would also part. The same applies to the allergens and infections, including those caused by the vaccination.

Chapter 4

The birth

The position

The deliveries are for several years in a manner that is far from being the one introduced by Mother Nature. Today, everything must be done quickly. They do not even take the time to live childbirth normally and as it should be. "Nothing is used to run, it must be based on point!" (Jean de La Fontaine)

Give Birth lying on the back may disrupt the oxygen supply in the fetus, since the weight of the uterus will crush the vessels which feed the blood flow. In the past, women gave birth to their knees, crouched or standing to facilitate the muscular work. What animal puts the bottom lying on the back? Do you know?

The nature does not like to be the thwarts. No cases of autistic child would not have been reported of a baby born at home by a midwife without medical intervention or pharmaceutical. A difficult birth would leave traces in the body and the psyche. The child is modeled by its passage.

The rupture of the waters

Some forms of autism may be related to a trauma of birth. The increase in the rate of use of the techniques of tripping of the work during the births corresponds strangely with the increase in the rate of autism. Women who give birth are not well enough informed about the risks incurred by the use of certain practices.

The breakdown of the water using a hook for cause or accelerate the work already initiated can disrupt the flow of blood to the head of the baby and pass the umbilical cord before his head, raising the risk of strangulation. This method increases the pain of contractions that, becoming intolerable in many cases, request to have recourse to the epidural anesthesia.

The Epidural Epidural ()

Some women who give birth receive a epidural anesthesia to decrease the pain of the contractions. It is a drug anesthésiante which would be a derivative of cocaine and which is directly injected into the nervous system the mother by a needle between two vertebrae at the bottom of the spinal column. This would prevent the women of Push properly when of contractions that they cannot even feel. The epidural anesthesia would slow down the work, which is simultaneously increase the need to have recourse to the use of the pitocin in order to raise the frequency and the intensity of the contractions.

"The epidural decreases the secretion of oxytocin or stops its normal increase during the work."[12] The cessation of pain is also lower the natural production of endorphin and adrenaline which is necessary during the final expulsion of the fetus out of the body of the mother. In addition, the muscles of the pelvic floor are numb by the epidural anesthesia. They can therefore not guide the head of the baby in the good position, which requires the use of forceps or of the suction cup with all the risks that this represents. Outbreaks less effective would also increase the recourse to cesarean section. The epidural anesthesia would cause sometimes a cardiac arrhythmia thus depriving the baby of blood and oxygen. The fever that can cause the epidural anesthesia in the mother may also cause brain damage in children. This medicine can cross the barrier of the placenta and reach the baby who is more vulnerable to the toxic effects. The new-born has more difficulties to extract the drugs than an adult. Since the latter s store in tissues such as those of the brain, this can cause fetal toxicity, an alteration of the central nervous system and cardiac abnormalities. The epidural anesthesia may disrupt the neurological functions of the baby as well as his respiratory rate during its first few hours of life.

The modification of the chemistry of the brain of the new-born form the basis of human behavior. Babies who have been exposed to the epidural anesthesia would become less skilled and more slow. Of the children born of a mother Rhesus (O Negative) who received the epidural anesthesia would have had by the result of the difficulties in normal stages of development. The everything would be derived from what is called a combination of risk factors.

The pitocin (oxytocin)

Oxytocin is a hormone that is found in mammals. It would be extracted from the pituitary gland of the beef for the manufacture of the pitocin. Yet, we are not of the cows. This artificial hormone is administered to women to increase the contractions, which would prevent the natural hormones to do their job effectively.

Where s stores any this secretion of hormones unnecessary and in surplus? Or what turns? This hormone a-t-it a role to play in the fact that it is boys who are more often with autism that the girls? The boys are they more sensitive to a hormonal imbalance? Hormones play a role in the process of detoxification. The estrogen would prevent the organization to get rid properly the heavy metals and other toxins. The boys would therefore have more difficulties to clean their system. In addition, if it is true that the pitocin would contain a substance similar to one found in pesticides and knowing that these can cause of neurological disorders, it is not surprising that this drug is equally toxic.

The hypothesis of a link between the pitocin and autism had attracted the attention of the media following the publication, in 1998, a study that state of an increase in the rate of autistic children born of a childbirth caused the pitocin. Some researchers then assumed that exposure to high rates of oxytocin at birth could increase the susceptibility to develop autism by decreasing of oxytocin receptors in the developing brain.[13]

There may be delayed effects, therefore in the long term, on the neurological development of children exposed to this medication. The drugs taken during the birth are imprisoned in the brain of the baby, which can change the speed of maturation of the brain cells, the position of these, their ability to exercise of the functions, the connection between their circuits and the speed of the nervous influx. The migration of neurons along the fibers would be modified by the change of the chemical composition of normal brain in full period of rapid development.

The alterations in the pace of the normal development of the brain cells create bad connections between the nerve fibers, which can lead to permanent damage during the hours following the birth. The brain of the fetus is much more vulnerable to the drug intoxication. The levels are higher among the child as in the Mother given its inability to extract as quickly as in the adult.

On the note of the manufacturer of the oxytocin, it would be written this: "maternal deaths due to episodes of high blood pressure, bleeding meningeal, rupture of the uterus, death of the fetus, the brain damage Permanent of the child due to various causes have been associated with the use of drugs ocytocines by parental track for the induction of labor." We also highlight other adverse effects such as permanent damage to the central nervous system, a Poisoning of amniotic fluids and cardiac arrhythmias. The decline in blood pressure in the mother affects the blood supply to the baby the depriving of oxygen.

The Contractions too strong and too long raccourciraient the availability of oxygen to the brain of the fetus. The abnormalities of the heart rate of the baby would create a fetal asphyxia. The baby deprived of oxygen at birth will therefore damage to cells of different organs of the body and, especially, to the brain. The considerable decrease in the oxygen supply in the brain of the

Nascent baby will impact on its development. Therefore, the perinatal asphyxia of the Newborn could be one of the causes of autism.

When the pitocin triggers heart rhythm abnormalities in the baby while it is still in the womb of its mother, it is difficult to believe that it could not be the origin of disturbances mental and physical damage caused by anoxia, which is a lack of oxygen at birth. These contractions, which would not be produced nor by the natural hormones in the baby or by those of the mother, could lead to a trauma of birth because the child is expelled out of the uterus without that his mother neither he are ready. This fetal distress is caused by the violent contractions that do not follow the natural rhythm of the mother or the unborn child. This creates a stress on both the body of the mother than on that of the child.

The oxytocin causes contractions much more violent and painful that natural contractions, requiring the use of the epidural anesthesia to decrease the suffering. A drug is therefore used to counter the undesirable side effects of the other, and vice versa.

"The marriage of epidural and pitocin, all of which two can cause abnormalities of the heart rate of the baby, reflects a fetal distress, markedly increases the risk of birth op (forceps, suction unit) or cesarean section."[14] In addition, the pitocin and the epidural anesthesia would lead to a compression in the skull of the baby. Interfere in the pace of the birth would prevent a good relationship between the expansion and the contractions of the pelvis of the mother of the same as those of the plates of the skull of the baby. This lack of coordination and synchronization between the pace of the mother and that of the Child requires the use of forceps and vacuum. Drugs shall submit the fetus to pressures enormous cranial. This pressure on the brain and on the cranial nerves would jeopardize the development of the central nervous system.

The frequency and the intensity of the contractions caused artificially do not arrive to dilate more the cervix. Other Surgical Interventions and pharmaceuticals is necessary. A veterinarian has said: "I do not even want to do this to the bitches who put down!" Is this the combination and the interaction between these two drugs that can trigger a certain form of autism?

There are data involving autistic disorders with the use of an artificial hormone that is given to pregnant women to cause or accelerate the work. It [the doctor Eric Hollander] has noticed that 60% of patients with autism in his clinic had been exposed to the drug. The material published by the World Health Organization

26

also notes an association between the use of pitocin and autistic disorders.[15]

This has been disputed by Health Canada. Not surprising! And yet, the terbuline, a neurotoxin in the same way as the pesticides that are manufactured on the basis of organophosphates, would be suspected to be part of the causes that can act as a trigger of autism. "The terbuline (terbutaline) is used as the provocateur of contractions at the end of the pregnancy. A neonatal study on laboratory rats has demonstrated brain abnormalities of fetuses of young rodents treated to the terbuline."[16]

The increase in the use of methods of birth modern with artificial interventions, mechanical, medical and pharmaceutical strangely corresponds to the increase of autism. Among the other disorders that are associated with the pressure on the skull and the body of the baby, we find: repeated ear infections, paralysis of the brain, episodes of seizures, dyslexia, learning difficulties, hyperactivity, behavioral disorders, of strabismus (eye Croche) and attention deficit, an evil of society!

But this is not all. The oxytocin would play a role in social relations in animals and would promote the commitment mother-child. It is known that the hormonal fluctuations in humans can influence the mood and behavior. In addition, oxytocin injected would interfere in the skills of breastfeeding delaying its first contact "mouth-nipple". These children have also often of the difficulty to suckle. Hormonal changes in the mother would make the availability of its milk more difficult, where could come a certain form of nutritional deficit. Some children with autism have a deficit in oxytocin which is caused by the use of artificial hormones blocking the production of natural hormones.

The anoxia

A child who was born in having missed of oxygen to the cells must follow the sessions in hyperbaric chamber, a treatment which seems to bear fruit for some children in the short and medium terms. This therapy would be effective to reduce inflammation. Then, why parents must they pay astronomical sums of money to repair the errors caused by the professionals of the Health?

The forceps

The use of forceps risk of move the bones of the skull and create bleeding in the brain.

Research conducted by a éthologiste and his wife on the autism have highlighted a number of factors likely to foster the Autism: install forceps, birth under anesthesia, resuscitation to the birth, triggering of the work... A high number of children born as a result of these practices are with autism. A more recent study on 184 children with autism highlights a triggering of the work of the delivery at the time of their birth in an average of 23 per cent of the cases studied.[17]

How many women have given birth with the use of strong methods and cruel, and how many of them have had a child with autism? What is of the physicians want to tell just by: "Your Child Is came to the world with autism!"?

The Sensory Defenses

It is very likely that a child who is suffering physically and mentally to his birth is the world very offensive and develops defense mechanisms to protect themselves, for example the downturn on itself, the loss of the desire to communicate with his entourage and the refusal to tame its environment. The child would seek to regain its uterine comfort by the regression. His behavior could well be a sign of disapproval by report to the way things were held. It has removed all the possibilities of well start in life. It is a false start.

An occupational therapist has said that a difficult birth can cause sensory defenses. This would be a way to protect themselves from a world that the child has found little welcoming. This is why some women want to have recourse to the kinésie to relive a normal delivery and a birth less traumatic for their child in order to keep a souvenir positive of this time. Is that what the hyper or the hyposensibilité in some children with autism would come from a difficult birth?

Chapter 5

The Dodo on the back

The syndrome of the flat head

Plagiocephaly, which is the flattening of the posterior part of the head of the baby, is also known under the term of the syndrome of the flat head. It is not only an aesthetic problem, since this could lead, in the long term, to the psychological and social.

The current custom of the "Dodo on the Dos" is part of a world-renowned program because of the specialists would have said that this position could prevent sudden infant death syndrome, although this sudden death can be caused by several other factors including the vaccination. This position would have the legacy much more serious than those planned. During that it attempts to save the life of one or two children at the national level, this position would lead to a delay in the development among millions of other children. Is it worth it?

A recent study [...] in fact reveals that the new-born babies who sleep on their backs acquire more slowly some motor skills keys, by comparison with those who sleep on the belly. However, limit the ventral position from infants to only phases of awakening would result in a delay in the development of the engine. The implications are no less important.[18]

The Dodo on the back Prevents children to use their fingers, hands, wrists, elbows and arms to raise in order to return. These children have more difficulty away their torso of the soil in taking on their hands when they are on the belly in the period of awakening. They have not had the chance to develop enough musculature of their neck, their backs and their buttocks, which makes them lose their mobility and the control. This would also negatively affect the development of the traction of the joins, since the passage of the nerve messages from the brain to muscles was not stimulated early enough. The hypersensitivity of the hands could well be one of these negative consequences.

Be lying on the belly would promote the development of the gross motor skills as well as the manual dexterity. This position would contribute to the development of the reactions of balance that lie at the basis of the maintenance of the position sitting and standing. The child will more quickly to roll, to crawl and walk at four legs of an autonomous manner. Babies who sleep on the back are to walk much later that the babies who slept on the belly in the past.

The child thus passes by above essential steps that must be followed to ensure a normal development. It would thus increase the risk of developing a delay early engine, which would explain why some children begin to walk much later than average and that others do the same on the end of the feet.

Some children spend walking on the knees to the upright position without having to go through the phase of crawl on the ground and walk to four legs. A problem of balance and coordination to be at the origin, since a part of the brain would not happen to develop the following skills as long as it would not have saved the prerequisites as acquired. It is thus that a delay of the walk can cause at the same time a delay of the development of the language, since these two areas would be in the same place in the brain. The infant which remains quite long periods lying on the belly goes through all the steps of the normal development (crawling, rolling, walk four-legged, dragging on the knees and stand up). To prevent choking by gastric reflux possible, the best position for the sleep would remain on the side.

Of the brain cells may have been damaged by the crash of the behind the head, which can result in various disorders.

It [the plagiocephaly] produces for the cuts and the tensions, particularly in the nervous system of the cerebellum and the pituitary gland, a deviation of the Jaw likely, among others, to harm the suction and to breastfeeding, the adverse impact on the vision of the baby, its balance, its coordination, his body schema, his sleep, his mood and even its growth.[19]

The negative consequences could even have an impact on the hand-eye coordination, one of the characteristics of the pervasive developmental disorders.

As I said at the beginning, factors other than those directly related to the position of the sunset on the back in a period of sleep are responsible of the Sudden infant death syndrome. It may be, among others, abnormalities of the immune system. Since the sudden infant death syndrome is higher among boys than girls, do you not see a link with autism? If the pervasive developmental disorders are triggered by the vaccination, there is no doubt that the latter could also be responsible for the Sudden infant death syndrome.

Chapter 6

Visual pollution and sound

We live in a world where coexists pollution in all its forms. There is the noise of large towns and cities and household appliances. All consist of waves of high or low frequency. We are also bombarded with images and "Flash" lights, either those of the screens or of car headlights without forgetting those cameras.

A psychologist had written an article which stated that the television could cause of autistic symptoms. The brain would be too stimulated by the various tones and the short sequences of images, which would result in the child in an unreal world and abnormal. The circuits between neurons would develop and would connect otherwise at that time. The constant noise can interfere with the interior monologue of the child where he would learn to a specific period of time the way to find solutions to the problems. Yet, in the book everything is played before 6 years, Dr. Dodson said that the television can contribute to the development of the language.

According to studies, the rate of autism would have increased at the same time that sales of TVS, DVDS, video games, computers, cellular phones and other notebooks of the same kind.

The polls already showed that there is a rate of autism higher among children who live in the regions rainy. However, these watch more television than those who live in sunny areas. The researchers have also found a relationship between the number of people with autism and the number of subscribers to cable in some regions.[20]

Sedentary stay does not favor the psychomotor development. It is by playing that one learns to explore while living of sensory experiences necessary for development. According to me, what is the most harmful, it is the lack of physical exercise that could lead to disorders of the development on the plan of the fine motor skills and comprehensive. It would also prevent the child to develop in exploring its environment while allowing his brain to store information from its five meaning and to be able to deal with them. This is not looking at television for hours that he can develop his imagination by the game. It is necessary to go outside and take in fresh air.

The TV could be detrimental to a child with a tendency toward the autism in the preventing of having social interactions with the other. It should not be forgotten that the practice of physical exercise contributes to a better oxygenation of the cells and the sweating helps to excrete the toxins from the body.

Television could therefore have a responsibility in the hyperactivity and attention deficit including behavior disorders and learning difficulties. The child might not find the teacher as interesting as a screen where many things move quickly while making the noise.

"The computer screens and television reduces the level of melatonin (a hormone that controls the biological rhythms of sleep and of sleep) in the blood, which can contribute to early puberty."[21] melatonin could therefore have an impact in the development or the triggering of the autism, since several of these children suffer from a sleep disorder. Since that television exists, the people are inclined to lie much later than before. A good sleep helps to strengthen the immune system, thus helping to fight infections. The great sleepers have a immune system more efficient. The animals who sleep many have less infections viral, bacterial and parasitic diseases.

The insomnia therefore increases the vulnerability to diseases. The immune system plays a major role also to the detoxification. A good sleep aid the body to make the vacuum of the negative and full of positive. Therefore, television could influence the functions of the immune system.

Chapter 7
The Vaccines

Especially do not affect (Hippocrates)

"The one who does not know that what he is doing is wrong and that the fact when the same is an ignorant or a fool; But the one who knows that what he is doing is wrong and that the fact when the same is a criminal!" (Conference of Montreal, 2009).

"Schools of Medicine have a long and sordid history of Corporal toward the bearers of new ideas, particularly if these innovative ideas belie beliefs long cherished, such as those that vaccines are benign and do not cause any wrong."[22] If a doctor says that he did not know, despite all the information that travels on this subject, that vaccines can cause autism and other autoimmune diseases, chronic and degenerative diseases, it is as if he said: "I pulled on someone with a rifle, but I was not aware that there was a bale inside it."

The ignorance is contagious

Why vaccines do they not all children with autism? I spoke earlier of genetic predisposition and environmental impacts. Not everyone reacts the same way. We are all different. Here is an example: if we give the same amount of alcohol to different people, they will not become all drunk at the same time. Some fall asleep, others will become hyperactives, hysterical, euphoric, aggressive, violent, depressed, passive or suicidal.

The same goes for the vaccines since the immune system is different from one person to the other. Some suffer from a disability immune. It was therefore wrong to believe that vaccines are suitable for all the world.

If this vaccine does not render such a person with autism, however, there is the risk that the latter will suffer later of Attention Deficit, hyperactivity, depression, diabetes, Alzheimer disease or cancer. It all depends on where the heavy metals and other harmful substances will lodge.

Mother Nature has not designed as well

Everything that goes counter to the nature we plays of the towers and we falls above. Since when caught us several diseases at the same time? The epidemics have emerged one at a time in the history of humanity.

The skin is the most important system of defense. Usual, the diseases penetrate the interior of our organization by a natural entry as the respiratory tract or digestive tract. This is not normal to receive Viruses and bacteria accompanied of toxic products by the skin, directly in a muscle of the arm to then find themselves in the blood stream. The skin is as a barrier: it protects us against the invaders. And we break this natural protection in the crossing with needles.

It is quite normal that the body would also react badly to this assault unusual. How can he combat these diseases all at the same time in addition to all the toxic substances which accompany them? Our immune system we imposes its limits; it is not a super hero.

The Placebo Effect

Doctors would believe much in the Placebo Effect of the evils of unknown provenance or psychosomatic. Vaccines have made their appearance at the same time as the natural decline, that is to say the free fall and predictable in the life cycle of the virus and bacteria related to large epidemics. This is the reason for which the great of this world believe in their effectiveness, then that it would be that of a placebo effect.

Why receive as much of vaccines while our living conditions and hygiene are improved? Is it normal, with the increase of vaccines and drugs, that people are more sick that once the point of overflowing the emergency clinics, and the hospital centers? Is it possible that the Vaccines (and drugs), instead of halting the disease, have created new? Do we want to really exchange measles against autism, leukemia, diabetes and cancer? According to a new study, the measles virus would protect against cancer; In response, pharmaceutical companies would have suddenly invented a false measles epidemic in order to revaccinated children in all the schools. They claimed that this epidemic would have appeared as a result of the decrease of this vaccine, but I believe that it would be rather an alert due to their decrease in income. "The cancer was virtually unknown before the vaccination, and I have never seen a single among an unvaccinated person."[23]

The vaccines contain 50 per cent of mercury, attenuated viruses, bacteria died, and chemical toxins such as aluminum, formaldehyde and detergents... It would be difficult to believe that pieces of microbes artificially mitigated or genetically modified organisms injected could prevent a disease. It is as if we said that he must give small casual rape to children in the aim to prepare them for a possible rape without risking to hurt physically and mentally.

The effectiveness of vaccines would never have been proven scientifically, only financially since they would lead to huge profits. I asked my veterinarian the reason for which he had as much of reminders of vaccines for the domestic animals. He answered me that it is because they are not even certain that they ensure a really immunity. He added that the live virus were withdrawn from the

33

vaccines for animals, because they felt that it was too dangerous for them.

The auto-immunity... self-destruction!

During the last 20 years, we have seen an increase in autoimmune diseases, which is strangely to an increase of vaccinations.

Stimulate in a manner as aggressive and not very natural defense mechanisms may cause relatively serious consequences. The vaccination would be the more coarse of errors in any medical history of humanity. I have even heard an American doctor say the following words at a conference on autism given to Montreal in 2012: "vaccines and antibiotics are an insult to the intelligence medical." The antibiotics would not contribute to strengthen the immune system; on the contrary, they attack and weaken it.

The formulants would "overshoot" the immune system in the offensive. That is what they call the "Stimulate"! I called it the "tip". After being distort, panic installs and seizes Him. This abnormal activation would trigger an autoimmune response pushing to produce antibodies against its own cells. Or well, it is frozen by fear and does not react not knowing where to give the head, because this overexcitement would prevent to differentiate which is itself of what is not. This disorder would attack its own organization as if it was a foreign body. It is a little like an animal female who will eat its small in the aim of protecting them. He does not know to distinguish between what is dangerous and what is not.

The auto-immunity can be caused by a infectious aggression of viral origin and chemical, therefore vaccine. Vaccines and viruses in too big quantity create a stress on the immune system. And this is not the whole world that reacts well to this assault and the stress they cause. The genetic inheritance could also shape a defensive response abnormal. The autism could well be a defect of the immune system which is often the result of an environmental trigger.

The human being will destroy itself (Albert Einstein)

The squalene is an adjuvant that would now be used in some vaccines including that against the flu. In the normal state, it is found in some fatty foods and oily. Normally, it enters the body through the oral routes for shelter in the bodies which have the greatest need as the brain. In the vaccines, it would come from the oil of shark which could well be the cause of new allergies to fish. If the vaccine causes an immune response against one of its components, as it may be the case of squalene, he therefore risks to attack also all the parts of the body that contain including the brain.

If the immune response is very strong, the adjuvant can further damage the brain, causing a deficit in essential fatty useful for its proper functioning. The adjuvant can galvanize the response of the immune system and thereby result in a reaction self-defeating against his own squalene.

Researchers are more and more convinced that the vaccination could be responsible for the weakening of the immune system and would be the cause of a aberrant immunity which, in turn, would trigger allergies. These allergies are not visible (skin rash), but they are manifested by food intolerances which can in turn lead to any form of neurosis, of psychosis, behavior disorder or dysfunction of the brain.[24]

If the culture of a vaccine is done on the spinal cord of animals, this could cause a response auto-immune against the own nervous system of an individual in which he was inoculated. If a vaccine is grown on the bile of beef, the attack auto-immune function may occur against its own gallbladder and cause a malfunction of the liver. If the virus has been multiplied on an embryo aborted, antibodies may occur against the fetus of a pregnant woman and cause a miscarriage, more commonly called "Spontaneous abortion". The albumin human and animal used in the manufacture of vaccines can also ensure that the human being who the attack receives its own albumin. In this case, adjuvants and additives can trigger of autoimmune diseases. The immune system would develop antibodies against its own cells.

An abnormal immune response ensures that the immune system reacts against its own organs and creates antibodies "specific body" against itself. In the case of autoimmune reactions in autism, the organ in question is mostly the brain. However, the digestive organs, especially the intestine, can also be targeted.[25]

Adjuvants or opponents: allies or enemies?

"Adjuvants to a single vaccine can cause a immune boost that can last up to two years."[26]

The body could consider the immunization act as inappropriate. Indeed, since the substances injected implement an immune response which is not natural, the defense system can therefore trigger an allergy to vaccines or to one or several of its components, which could explain the anaphylactic shock in the case of the Sudden infant death syndrome or any other form of unexplained death. "The Stabilizing gelatin found in food products and vaccines as the MMR (measles, mumps, rubella vaccine) has been involved in the anaphylaxis."[27]

The bovine gelatin in vaccines could well be at the origin of allergies to dairy products including the beef protein. The babies would be the most sensitive to the toxicity of vaccines and their chemical components as they would receive, at a time when their immune system is not fully developed, the same amount as an adult would not even be able to tolerate. The overload of the immune system would be at the origin of a beginning of intoxication. The autism could well be a form of poisoning of different natures.

What will we eat tomorrow?

Since vaccines are grown on heifers or still on of contents dairy, it goes without saying that the immune system would develop antibodies against the bovine protein that we consume orally by the result, triggering at the same time the allergies (including the one to the casein) and Intolerance to lactose. The flu vaccine could trigger an allergy to eggs, since the latter is inoculated on chicken embryos. We do not eat when not even this food by the skin of the arm! Of the people would have developed an allergy to eggs while they have never eaten. Look for the Error! What happens to people who will no longer be able to consume cereals, or dairy products or meat?

Cruelty to animals or crime against humanity?

Since vaccines are grown on animal protein, millions of animals, fetus and eggs are sacrificed for the manufacture of vaccines during that there are still people who are suffering and dying of hunger throughout the world. Indeed, in both poor and rich countries, there are children who do not eat breakfast before going to school and who do not eat to their hunger. There is also a risk that the human being is done contaminate by diseases from other animal species.

The virus of the bovine diarrhea was detected in approximately 30% of a human population studied even if the latter had no physical contact with infected animals. It is recognized that these viruses, passing the species barrier, can mutate, recombine between them or to reactivate latent viruses. New strains of viruses have been isolated in human cells and they showed similarities with bovine strains.[28]

An attack against-indicated

There is a link between some viruses and autism.

When an animal is vaccinated, the rate of inflammatory agents is increasing considerably in his brain. This creates a stimulation of the immune system. The principal cells of the brain are agitated quickly, as if the order had been given to fight an enemy. It results in several days or even weeks, inflammation of the brain is reflected by the agitation, irritability, insomnia, fatigue, a feeling of being in the fog.[29]

A brain in full development may suffer greater damage that if he had reached a stage of maturity. When viruses enter the brain, the immune system has an alert level high. Viruses and bacteria would result in an immune response that is directed to the brain tissues taking the central nervous system as the enemy. This would disrupt the development central nervous.

Environmental factors such as viruses, chemicals, toxins, bacteria and parasites cause a malfunction and a disruption of the immunity that trigger an attack against a brain tissue causing of disorders neuro-immunological which lead to autism, since it is the brain that manages and directs the immune response. Therefore, the immune system overloaded with applications believes that the attack comes from the brain; it is for this reason that it response to his turn. An atypical infection of measles can develop a response auto-immune directed against the myelin in the brain.

The auto-immunity resulting from a virus and directed against the myelin of the brain could hinder the anatomical development of neural pathways among children. A reaction auto-immune affecting the brain structures, in particular the myelin sheath, would play an important role on the plan of the Neurological alterations found in people with autism. In addition, a immune aggression, as a result of an infection or a vaccination, could cause "gaps" or of small changes in the myelin sheath. The latter could finally alter permanently the higher mental functions, i.e. learning, memory, communication, social interactions.[30]

Several factors are involved in the emergence of autoimmune diseases; first, the microbes whose virus can bind to a gene and modify the immune response. They could therefore act as mutagenic agents. We have seen previously the role of environmental impacts in the genetic mutation.

There would also be a greater production of antibodies among boys than girls because of hormones, which would explain why there are more boys than girls with autism.

Let us take a drink to our health

The vaccines would be composed of a toxic cocktail worthy of the largest revenue of witchcraft. Here is the list of ingredients that could be found in some vaccines: Albumin human or animal, aluminum, sodium borate (insecticide, rat-poison "Biorat"), mercury, sorbitol, silicone, aspartame, beta proprio lactone, formaldehyde (carcinogenic), Bovine gelatin or swine, gentamycin (antibiotic), polymyxin, monosodium glutamate, glutaradelhyde, lactose, latex (allergen), neomycin (an antibiotic), monosodium glutamate (hyperactivity), phenol (antifreeze), polysorbate, squalene, bovine serum, Ammonium sulphate; viruses and bacteria, some of which are genetically modified on cells made carcinogens, animal from which the dog, the cat, rabbit, the monkey, the sheep, pork, duck, the hamster, the chicken, the mouse, the cow; of fetal calves aborted or of human embryos as well as chicken embryos that carry all of the diseases specific to Their species and whose particles of their DNA could change our own genetic background. To think that this can give us health, it is a little to believe in the magic.

The bovine serum may be the bearer of the mad cow disease or CJD, the chickens are carriers of the avian influenza virus and the African green monkeys, of HIV. The toxins that emit Viruses and bacteria create tumors in animals. Was there as much of cancer cases before the advent of vaccines to massive dose?

The vaccination, a form of dictatorship

In the past and still today, dictators have been arrested, imprisoned, tried and executed for having committed crimes against humanity. When will stop this massacre? I am not a doctor, so I can allow myself to say all top this that many physicians believe any bottom by fear of losing their license to practice and especially the beautiful flowered retirement bride who goes with the purchase of the silence. Why doctors refuse-they to vaccinate their own children?

Nobody is questioned on the possibility of recombination of the virus between them to give birth to new diseases when a fragmentation of virus is unit to another in order to complement each other.

In the case of the MMR vaccine, it is of live virus that could wake up after having been somewhat poorly stunned. It might then be that viruses asleep, fragmented or mitigated are not combated by the immune system that there would see that that is no danger, since they would be incomplete, but that this would not prevent the virus to develop a part of the disease in the form of associated symptoms. The immune system could be more concerned to combat the chemical components and toxic of vaccines and would thus pass the virus or then, could not tackle to only one at a time, it would flee the other. The attenuated viruses defy as well the defense system, they would the shelter and could regain their virulence in another environment where the immune system has got rid of the formaldehyde that prevented them to express themselves.

"Since the 1960s, scientists knew that an attenuated virus may, in rare circumstances, mutate and regain its virulence, but this is only in 2000 that they realized that they could transmit the disease between the people."[31]

New diseases can therefore appear by recombination and by viral mutation.

The absence of a link between the MMR vaccine and autism would never have been scientifically demonstrated in an absolute way and, especially, credible otherwise than by the studies made by the pharmaceutical companies that manufacture the vaccine or by private organizations but subsidized by the latter. If we knew all of the reports which have been modified or kept secret! We must understand that all those who are of the clinical studies the font in function of what they are trying to prove and that all data is not corresponding are put aside, are hidden or are not taken into consideration, in the hope that the population will never account. They can therefore even change the statistics in their favor.

"The interactions between vaccines have not been seriously studied under the angle of the repeated vaccinations and immune system potentially fragile."[32] Before the marketing of vaccines, the observation periods were often too short to predict the neurological sequelae in the medium and long terms. Only the short-term side effects have been observed.

Nightmare, illusion or reality?

The presence of the measles virus in the intestines represents an inadequate response and unexpected of a weakened immune system. The latter would cause the inflammation in the intestines and to the brain. Research, for which the results would not have been spread to the great day, demonstrated that the MMR (measles, mumps, rubella) caused colitis and digestive disorders. In the intestines of some children with autism, researchers would have found the presence of traces of attenuated viruses from the vaccine against measles. Knowing that the measles virus can cause inflammation of the brain, there would therefore be a link between the intestines and the brain. This would explain why the cranial perimeter of some children with autism appeared to be wider than that of children expressed normal.

We have seen an interesting correlation between the measles antibodies and the auto-immunity directed against the brain tissue, revealed by the presence of auto-antibodies directed against the protein of basis of the myelin, which suggests a link between the measles virus and the auto-immunity among people with autism. The component anti-measles patients of the combined vaccine measles-mumps-rubella could be in question. Therefore, we believe that the anti component measles-of the MMR vaccine could trigger a reaction auto-immune in autistic children.[33]

The measles in itself can cause inflammation of the brain, a sensitivity to the light which is a Stroke autism; encephalitis, which are an inflammation of the membrane surrounding the brain that can cause seizures, as is the case in some children after vaccination; of mental retardation or a sudden death. Measles would also infections of ears. "The major complications of measles are the respiratory superinfections such that a purulent rhinitis, pneumonia, laryngitis, pharyngitis, a otitis or bronchitis. Sometimes, measles can cause encephalitis or meningitis (neurological complication)."[34]

Rubella could also create encephalitis and meningitis, even if it is only in rare occasions, as well as the brain lesions. This would also explain the fact that a certain percentage of vaccinated children develops autism as well as the immune weaknesses in some individuals. If the one can die of rubella, it is not surprising that this vaccine can also cause a sudden death. Rubella is a disease which can create delays and mental illness, and the growth disorders. Do you not see there the similarities with autistic traits? How can we inject at the same time three viruses, each of which is likely to cause of dementia? The fact that this is not all the persons affected in the past by these diseases which have suffered from dementia as a result of an infection would explain why this are not all children who become with autism after having received injections.

Cult or obsession absurd?

If the inflammation occurs to bodies other than the brain (as the pancreas), c is the diabetes that will develop. The mumps also affect the hearing and can make deaf. This is why children with autism do not seem to hear. This would therefore not just the content of vaccines that would be harmful, but also the effect of these injections on certain parts of the body.

If the vaccines were really effective, the antibodies would be ready to go to the attack following the many reminders of vaccines. But this is not what is happening because of the virus involved have been found in the bone marrow and the intestines. They would have managed to circumvent the immune system.

"Autism has been multiplied by 30 between 1978 and 1999, the United States and in London. This corresponds to the vaccination campaigns in these two countries. The chance does not exist."[35] There has been an increase in the rate of autism in the countries where the vaccination became mandatory. Before, the MMR vaccine was administered separately and at a distance at a time where the vaccines were that of 8 instead of 40 as would be the case today, then that our living conditions and hygiene have curbed propagations microbial and epidemics. Why is there no cases of autism in children who have never been vaccinated?

"Nobody has done the research to check if the exposure of infants to the vaccination as it is practiced is safe."[36] The child exposed too young to viruses of the measles, rubella and mumps may develop chronic diseases. A form of infant disability is attributable to neurological complications caused by infections, because the brain has its own immunity and therefore creates itself of inflammation. The brain and the immune system communicate together since the immune system works with the intestines; when those are swollen, the same thing occurs in the brain, and vice versa. We could call it a neurodevelopmental complication due to immunization. The autism would therefore be an autoimmune disease caused by vaccination. The MMR vaccine was injected to monkeys and those are become with autism. The fact to remove the existing formula of this vaccine would decrease the rate of new cases of autism.

The second Brain

The intestines are considered as the second brain, because they can operate independently. "The intestine is the second nervous system the more important after the brain."[37]

Millions of neurons are located along the digestive tract to check the functions related to the digestion as if it were a second independent brain. Secretin is equally present in the intestines that in the brain. It has a role to play in the intestinal permeability. This brings me to query on the similarity between the lesions in the brain, the myelin, and the porosity of the bowel. The intestines regulate the passage of nutrients through the mucous membrane while preventing harmful agents to penetrate in the blood and the poisoning. Destroy the intestinal membrane contributes to a blood poisoning. Intestinal hormones are therefore in direct communication with the blood system and some bodies related to the digestion. The intestinal system secretes of neurotransmitters identical to those found in the brain. It also produces 80% of immune cells. Tackle the immune system, is to address the intestines and the brain. Therefore, when things are not going well in the belly, that will not do well in the head. "Because neurotransmitters and neuromodulators of the brain are almost always also present in the intestine, drugs that act on the synapses in the brain are likely to have effects in the intestines."[38]

Antidepressants and other psychotic or neuroleptics could therefore create Gastrointestinal disorders or worse and thus influence the operation of the immune system. Of women who had taken antidepressants could then have an autistic child, the result of the secondary effects of the medication. And if the brain is poorly fed to cause gastrointestinal problems, other mental illnesses are added to the list.

"To have holes in the colon can make anxious and neurotic... Your intestine may make you crazy."[39]

A lost battle in advance

A mutation in a gene, which is responsible of the immunity, may result in damage to the capacity of the immune system to fight several infections. Viruses or bacteria, or toxic substances that they produce, can cause the failure of a gene. It could be a brain impairment by a virus paired with a failure of the immune system. An insufficiency of the functioning of the liver may be also responsible since it is he who manages the toxins from the body. Drugs can change the intestinal flora and at the same time the defense mechanisms. Therefore, a too large administration of drugs to the population can cause damage. The drugs are only hide the symptoms without never adjust the causes nor the evil at its source. Take drugs for life proves that they do not heal.

A failure would allow immune to a virus to attack the brain or cause an immune response against the latter. The inflammation of the brain which follows cause of neurological damage. A lack of oxygen to the brain and convulsions may result.

The brain of the fetus may be attacked directly if the mother has been vaccinated against measles shortly before conception or during her pregnancy. It could have an autistic child at birth.

Too much, it is too

Some children would not produce antibody to rubella due to an anomaly in their defense system or that of their mother, or because the vaccines are not a natural infection which is recognized by the system. The antibodies against measles are much higher among children with autism and children expressed normal, which demonstrates an immune response inadequate or excessive in some children which is certainly due to the inappropriate stimulation produced by aluminum present in the vaccine. In fact, the Aluminum extends the duration of immunity of a exaggerated way that may be spread over several months or years. This immune response comes from a reaction abnormal particularly against infection by a live attenuated virus.

"Some children with autism, for cause of a genetic anomaly affecting their immune system, cannot fight adequately some virus, even for forms mitigated."[40]

It was found in the intestines of 85 per cent of children with autism measles antibody affecting gastro-intestinal functions. A new form of intestinal inflammation has been discovered among children with autism, given the amount of white blood cells in their intestines. These elements are sufficiently credible to confirm a link between autism, the MMR vaccine and bowel disorders. Why does the government withdraws-t-it not the ROR until its security to be proven for all? The vaccines to unique strain would be more safe and effective as those to strain multiple. However, they would be more expensive. Save the money is more important than the health. If antibodies in the blood of the mother can bind to the brain of the fetus and cause damage, say that of the antibodies produced by the vaccines on the brain of children? In fact, too of antibodies would be associated with neurological disorders. "More and more neurological diseases appear to be related to a process auto-immune. Several disorders affecting the central nervous system and are characterized by the presence of auto-antibodies."[41]

The results of blood tests show an unusually high rate of antibodies in children with autism, which would prove that their immune system has actually been assaulted, disrupted and out of adjustment. The body then fight against its own immune defenses. All antibodies products in so little time and in industrial quantity would be considered by the body as invaders themselves and could then be seen as harmful and irritable. These antibodies irritants would also be dangerous for the brain of the fact of their too large number. They can even create brain lesions sometimes irreversible if the rate of antibodies is not reduced to time. The damage which are produced elsewhere in the body would lead to a delay of growth, including the pervasive development disorder.

The immune response as well shaken would send signals for the production of anti-antibodies, which would further weaken since it would be concerned to destroy what it has itself created. There is auto-antibodies, anti-antibody and antirécepteurs themselves, who would be directed against the serotonin.

"A Portuguese study has demonstrated the presence of antibodies in brain tissue of people with autism. The probable origin is the auto-immunity caused by environmental pollution."[42]

It is therefore of neuroimmune disorders since there is a resemblance between the auto-antibodies of the brain and the measles antibody found in the intestines. If auto-antibodies are attacking the organs or systems, the person could develop diabetes, arthritis, the hyper or hypothyroidism. If they are attacking the intestines, these become porous. If particles mysterious is found in the brain, it swell by an immune response inappropriate, which would trigger the production of antibodies against the neurons. There is therefore self-antibodies directed against the brain and other organs. The autism would therefore part of autoimmune diseases.

The antibodies would impede the chemical transmission at the level of the receivers. The presence of antibodies directed against the brain cells would prevent the nerve impulses to carry out adequate transmissions between the neurotransmitters. Auto-antibodies would also be directed against the blood vessels in the brain. A toxin present in the vaccines would separate the proteins of brain receptors, making ineffective the functioning of certain vitamins. The brain as well hungry lack of essential nutrients to function well.

A immune deficit makes vaccination inefficient, inadequate and dangerous. Autoimmune diseases develop especially among people who have followed an intensive immunization program.

Give me the oxygen

An eye or a corner of the mouth deviant are also due to a lack of oxygen caused by a blockage of blood more commonly known as a micro-vascular attack (cerebral).

The Vaccines cause a hyperreactivity of the immune system. Foreign products injected into the blood stream eventually clog, block. The road is therefore switched off for the red blood cells more small which should bring oxygen to the different organs. These particles that reach the brain disrupts or prevent the circulation of the blood, which can cause autism.[43]

The additives of vaccines would generate an immune response long and fast which would create blockages in the blood vessels, since the immune response is too strong. The same thing happens when one is prisoner of his car in a plug of movement or worse, in an accident. When the path is blocked, there is not always of detours possible. Those who escape them can take shortcuts. The production of antibodies is in too significant quantity; given that the white blood cells are larger and more numerous, they block the blood vessels and thus prevent the passage of red blood cells carry oxygen and nutrients, especially where the blood vessels are small as is the case in the brain. The blood clogged can no longer transport effectively the oxygen and the essential nutrients. A decrease of cerebral blood flow is associated with a form of dementia. Blockages in different receptors essential affect the language, to the attention, to the perception and sensations that can cause the dyslexia, the dysphasia, hyperactivity, the manic depression, chronic fatigue, schizophrenia, fibromyalgia, as well as tumors. The lack of oxygen prevents the brain to transmit the good information to muscles and organs.

When a cell is deprived of oxygen, she dies. It may be therefore that the intestinal porosity comes from the death of some cells precisely deprived of oxygen by vascular obstruction. If the brain is reached, this could explain the pervasive developmental disorders, as well as the increase in deficits of attention, of the difficulties of learning or diabetes if the component affected is the pancreas.

Before, the atmosphere contained 40% of oxygen; today, with the pollution and deforestation, it remains less than 20%. Nothing to contribute to a better health.

The battery is to earth

A deficiency of a nutrient weakens the immune system which is sometimes already out of adjustment. The nutrient status of the individual acts on the effectiveness of its immune system. The nutritional deficit also cause brain problems, since the brain has need of nutrients to function well. An exposure appropriate to the sun without protection during a short period when the rays are not at their maximum can prevent vitamin D deficiency which the receptors in the brain and nerve connections have both need. That is why of Depressed people need of brightness. In this case, the lack of sun could trigger a nutrient deficit leading to the autism. The sun creams detrimental to the production of vitamin D. The supply influences the brain functions and intestinal infections.

Among the other sources contributing to the depletion of defense mechanisms, one finds: the cleaning products, disinfectants, industrial products of tangible hygiene, food pushing with chemical fertilizers and pesticides, genetically modified organisms (GMOS), the chemical products used in the processing of food whose flavor

45

enhancers,, the dyes, the artificial flavors, preservatives, additives, the packaging of food in toxic materials such as plastic and aluminum, air pollution, molds of houses and ventilation systems.

For multiple infections can trigger of autoimmune diseases. The vaccines against hepatitis B, diphtheria, tetanus and pertussis would also be responsible, accomplices with the MMR vaccine and influenza. Imagine what can happen if a child receives all these vaccines on the same day. They can all cause epileptic seizures, meningitis and encephalitis.

If the pertussis vaccine is contraindicated in the case of neurological diseases, one could believe that it can cause the same kind of harm (or amplify the problem) especially if nobody is studying the field before the injections and if the parents or patients are not informed about the risks. The MMR vaccine would be contraindicated in the case of a family history of immune deficits, autoimmune diseases and allergies. But that takes this into account before to inject these microbes to someone? If Rubella can cause abnormalities of development, it is not surprising that there is an increase in pervasive developmental disorders.

When children are seized, enrhumés or grappling with a gastroenteritis, some autistic symptoms resurface more than usual, which would support the hypothesis that the immune system is involved in this phenomenon. There is a link between the central nervous system and the immune system. The disorders in one of these locations are reflected to other systems. The immune systems, nervous and digestive system are involved in autism. All the systems and bodies work in a team and not separately as the would believe many physicians. Holistic medicine recognizes that.

The drop that made the vase overflow

Inject too early several viruses at the same time in the body would destabilize the immune system that is not accustomed to such excessive invasions, especially when the latter is still immature. How can we expect to a perfect job of a system which has not reached its potential without even harm to its development and normal operation?

That the virus or bacteria are fragmented and weakened, dead, alive or mitigated in of formaldehyde, a substance toxic and carcinogenic, nothing prevents that children receive too large quantities much too early, without spacing or rest. The fragmentation of a virus could develop in a single aspect of the disease. The autism could well be a form of intoxication to viruses since some can even emanate from the toxins and harmful vapors in the body.

Studies have attempted to demonstrate that our system can eliminate the heavy metals such as mercury by the natural channels. The researchers would not have taken into consideration that the disorders of metabolism may affect some people who are more vulnerable than others. They claim that the defense system of the whole world works in the same way, at the same speed and with the same intensity, without considering the case where a person suffering from an immune deficiency. And yet, the doctors are well aware of the genetic differences individual.

A discount in question is required

This has taken How many time before to accept the theory of Galilee about the roundness of the Earth? How many children will they suffer in the name of profit before traveling to the obvious? Everyone knows the proverb saying that it is better to prevent than to cure.

It should be that any vaccination practice is regarded in the magnifying glass and passed to the comb end. It would be strongly recommended to exclude the use of live virus, eliminate all toxic substances including heavy metals and formaldehyde, not to use multiple vaccines, space each vaccine for several months and only for a single disease, not to give the first vaccine before the age of twelve months, since the child has received the antibodies which he has needed by the blood and breast milk, and immunize the population only against actual diseases which are really dangerous and that still exist in our time outside of laboratories, and especially if there is no effective treatment. The microbes should be introduced into the body by the natural channels, i.e. in the same way that we attraperait such disease. There is a need to study the field by checking the medical history of family and check if such individual can withstand the vaccine. If a person has a high rate of heavy metals in the blood, it is a sign of this disability; this would show that its system does not happen to detoxify. If the child has already the measles antibody that he has received by his mother, it is unnecessary that it receives this vaccine.

A vicious circle

The medicine of 10 000 years ago was based on the texture and on the scent of the stool. This practice of base has been lost of our days. Since the intestines work with the immune system, some virus and antibodies to set to the intestinal wall, causing the irritation followed by a inflammation that creates an anomaly of the intestinal mucosa. The number of bacteria and parasites and yeast is higher among children with autism who use of the injury of the mucosa to settle there.

The intestinal inflammation increases the permeability of the mucosa, because when it is inflated, it becomes thinner with more space between the cells. The mucosa, thus becoming porous, would pass of harmful substances and of food particles badly digested in the blood where they should never be there. Among the harmful particles which cross the intestinal mucosa become porous and who travel throughout the body by the circulation of the blood, are found certain proteins that may have an effect of opiate drug (strong) which act on some receptors causing behavioral disorders and learning. Intolerance to gluten contributes to the intestinal porosity since it disrupts the mechanism that governs the opening and closing of the doors of the intestinal mucosa which normally would pass the nutrients while retaining the toxins. The small doors would forget to close. In this case, gluten is responsible of intolerance to dairy products (casein) as well as other food allergies.

Immune disease and intestinal could be at the origin of neurological disorders, especially if one considers that vaccines and their components and destabilising and clog the defense mechanisms while irritating the intestines. The toxic particles from a feed containing chemicals such as pesticides are also set to the intestinal wall, the more damaging and thus allowing to parasites and yeasts to accede to and proliferate.

It should not be forgotten that this are the intestines which feed the brain as well as all other bodies. If they are damaged, how can they absorb the nutrients essential? If the blood is glutted with toxins, how can it carry vitamins and minerals? If the brain is poorly fed, how can it work well? A lack of vitamins, minerals, proteins and essential fats can disrupt the development and the functioning of the brain, and even more if the latter receives of toxic waste to the place. Regarding autism, it could be a form of blood poisoning.

In the attack

It induces the presence of antibodies against a food to the intestinal porosity. The immune system works hand in hand with the intestines. Approximately 76% of children with autism have the intestines porous, which explains a lot of things.

This is not normal to find tiny bits of food in some form in the blood. Not surprising that children with autism have as much of food allergies that can also cause inflammation in the intestines. In

48

addition, foods that are not well digested due to an immune reaction can irritate the mucosa of the intestines. Food allergies create inflammation to the esophagus, the throat and the rectum. "At least 70 per cent of our immune defenses are found in our intestines, then if, very early in the course of our life, the establishment of the intestinal flora is disturbed or is that inflammation is manifest, there may have major consequences on our ability to fight against infections and allergies."[44]

The intestinal flora shall inform the immune system and strengthens it. The intestines, the brain and the defense system are interrelated. Food allergies have therefore an impact on disorders concerning the behavior. Inflammation of the Esophagus cause of aggressive behaviors and waking at night. Food allergies can cause gastrointestinal disorders, gastro-enteritis, indigestion, of gastric reflux, ear infections, migraines, eczema and sinusitis; the whole plays on our moods and on our patience.

Of neurological disorders are linked to the hypersensitivity to gluten, to casein and soy, as well as to intestinal damage. "This becomes serious when, for example, the enzyme in question plays an essential role in the Degradation of gluten, of the casein or other foods. It is also for this reason that a food non-toxic which is not metabolised correctly becomes toxic to the body."[45]

We know that it is dangerous to give the chocolate to a dog. Since it has not the enzymes for the Digest, this can be a poison for him. Contract A virus to slow development may make changes of the immune response in the digestive system, which fact that some foods may be considered by the body as enemies.

Allergies and food intolerances would be from a immune provocation. The Army has become hypersensitive to the environment and the soldiers are become paranoid. Remove the food allergens would reduce the stress of the immune system and would decrease the rate of antibodies.

The power supply can also be perceived as a trigger component since too of carbohydrates (starches) in the power supply produces an enzyme that night to nerve cells. "Our mode of current nutrition promotes indeed a abnormal permeability of the small intestine and the training of food waste and hazardous bacterial which, crossing the expanded mesh of the intestinal mucosa, can cause immune reactions Adverse."[46]

Imagine of intestinal waste stroll in the brain and all the shots of circuit as this invasion can produce. It is like the fact of having parasites in the brain.

"Four thirty under for a buck"
Vaccines contain aluminum, another toxic heavy metal. It would replace the mercury. It would therefore be replaced a toxic heavy metal by another equally toxic. It is not fact that change the evil of place. The aluminum would be just as toxic to the brain that the mercury and lead. Its toxicity would increase especially when the kidneys of certain persons do not work well enough. It should then ask why they would use of aluminum in the treatment of dialysis.

"Young children can see administer up to 200 ug of aluminum by kilo in the space of one and the same visit to the pediatrician, 40 times the safety threshold admitted."[47] Among the signs of intoxication to the aluminum, would be: sudden alteration of intellectual capacity, problems with language, memory, socialization, muscle weakness, sleep disturbances, restlessness, instability, emotionality, headache, muscle pain, speech problems, visual deterioration, paralysis, anemia, problems of digestion, colitis, renal failure, mouth ulcers, difficulty in swallowing, fatigue, disorders of the bladder and incontinence, lesions on the abdominal organs, malfunction of the thyroid gland, thrombosis (blood clotting) that can lead to a sudden death by lack of oxygen, rheumatism, arthritis, hormonal dysregulation, sensitivity to Colds, confusion, depression, mood changes, suicidal thoughts, loss of the concept of time, red and irritated eyes, dizziness, feeling of drought in the throat and nose, pain in the chest in swallowing, change in appetite, alteration in the taste of food, waking at night with terrifying hallucinations, psychiatric problems various, cognitive deficit disorder, coordination, irrational reasoning, perception visuo-spatial altered, tremor, death by psychosis, cancer and blood poisoning. Do you not there several symptoms attributable to those of autism?

The autism was virtually unknown until 1943 when it was diagnosed and identified 11 months after that thimerosal, an adjuvant to basis of mercury, was introduced in the United States in the vaccines for infant, with other compounds to basis of aluminum.[48]

In vaccines, the Aluminum would be used to stimulate the immune system on a too long period. It is distressing to the point of no longer distinguish between what is dangerous and what is not. He would therefore to make antibodies against elements benign and harmless to the origin of the many food allergies. To trigger allergies in laboratory animals, it would suffice to mix the substance against which a reaction was desired with the aluminum salt such as the one that would be in vaccines. This heavy metal will increase the production of immunoglobulin. The vaccines against diphtheria, tetanus and pertussis would trigger also of allergies in laboratory animals. No cases of allergies has been observed in the human beings not vaccinated.

Who likes, vaccine little!

(Title of a book written by Swiss doctors)

The symbol of the traditional medicine is a snake turning around a pole. The vaccines could be in some way the bite of a venomous snake.

Mercury has long been considered a deadly poison. We would use again a mercury derivative, the thimerosal, entering as additive and conservation officer in vaccines injected for babies, children and adults, as well as the elderly with the "same dosage". The used vials for several people are what is called of multiple vaccines. The influenza would be part and they still contain thimerosal to prevent the vial to contaminate between the taken, because nothing would have found another to replace it. It would be too expensive to make vials to single dose.

The vaccines without thimerosal still contain mercury. An investigation by HAPI (Health Advocacy in the public interest) has demonstrated that the new vaccines (old vaccines recycled by filtering) so-called free from mercury contain when even this heavy metal with the addition of the aluminum. The pharmaceutical industry producer does not take the problem seriously. The filtering of mercury is inappropriate because the metal is fixed on the antigen of the protein in the vaccine.[49]

"Vaccine manufacturers have started to remove mercury from some injections to new-born Americans, while continuing to exhaustion old stocks of vaccines in mercury."[50] It seems that single-dose vaccines would contain more of thimerosal since a few years. However, some devices of manufacture would continue to be cleaned and disinfected with this product which can leave traces. That of hepatitis B in would contain yet, and it is suspected in the triggering of the autism.

Hepatitis B is a disease that is caught mainly by contact with the blood. The people most at risk would be the prostitutes, homosexuals, hemophiliacs, drug addicts, doctors, nurses and dentists. Why vaccinate infants against this disease? Just in case where the mother could be the carrier?! This allows pharmaceutical companies manufacturing this vaccine to enrich himself at the expense of the health of these children. Here are all the absurdity of the situation. "The new-born a danger extremely important, because their brain is not yet mature, the barriers between blood and brain are permeable and therefore more sensitive to the toxins."[51]

Slander or speculation?

The present medical system as well as the pharmaceutical companies would have tried to prove the non-toxicity of mercury which is nevertheless a deadly poison recognized since antiquity. What nonsense! Their deep convictions would have when even pushed to remove from some vaccines. If these people doubt of a possible link between vaccines and autism, why do withdraw they not of all vaccines? Answer: Because there would be a decline of autism and that they would be accountable to the population! Would they have fear of prosecution to the planetary scale? This is the reason for which they would maintain the mercury in the vaccine against influenza and strongly encourage it.

Number of researchers believe that the manufacturers have two reasons to oppose the total withdrawal of the thimerosal. The first is the lure of gain. The second, more important, is that they know that as soon as we will withdraw, the public will no longer be able to ignore the decline not only of autism, but also that of neurological disorder, attention deficit, hyperactivity, of language delay, which disrupt the school system since more than 15 years. This decline is already product in California, which was one of the first States to ban this poison.[52]

They would have then exported these vaccines to developing countries where s is developed the Autism. That Do they try to hide from the population? What interests do they try really to protect? The their? When the three-quarters of the hospitalizations are from the side effects of drugs and errors in medical acts, he must believe that this maintains jobs in place. Is it that the medical system is trying to protect the pharmaceutical industry is corrupt because it would Gifts to physicians in the aim to encourage them to prescribe and use their products which make people more sick without ever succeed to heal by camouflaging the symptoms by chemicals sometimes very toxic?

"Vaccines would have compounded a cellular disorder already existing - a disorder at the level of the mitochondria."[53] In this case, the vaccines would be aggressors who would trigger a predisposition. Therefore, they are responsible directly or indirectly, they are the cause, even if they trigger an anomaly which led to this disease. Why, if there is no danger with the vaccines, some governments protect they the pharmaceutical companies against any recourse? If the vaccines are not risky, why doctors do they now sign of papers to parents to absolve themselves of all responsibility in the case of adverse reactions? And why doctors refuse-they sign papers which are submitted to them by the parents worried that they take their professional responsibilities, financial and social issues in the case of adverse reactions in the short, medium and long terms?

There is little hope that the Tribunal decides in favor of the parents because the stakes are too enormous. If the court assigns compensation to the families of the victims, the pharmaceutical companies will not be immune from prosecution. The compensation will then be drawn from a fund established from a tax of 75 under by vaccine that the taxpayers already pay. However, if the Tribunal establishes a causal link, would be this only in one case, between autism and the presence of mercury in vaccines, the major pharmaceuticals could be the target of prosecutions at the planetary scale. In both cases, billions of dollars are at stake.[54]

One day, the orthodox medicine, conventional allopathic, regardless of the name given to it, will undergo a terrible scourge that it will greatly deserved because it will have caused. One day, their beautiful castle of cards will collapse. The population is already beginning to make them less and less confidence and to turn to natural medicines and soft. The Holistic medicine Environmental and will assume the responsibility and construct its empire on the ruins of the other.

"It is the dose makes the poison" (Paracelsus)

Mercury crosses the barrier of the placenta and would act as a neurotoxin amending the brain development of the fetus.

It is the accumulation of small quantities of mercury that is the greater risk to future mothers and their babies. In most chemical forms, mercury is a neurotoxin, which means it can cause damage to the brain and the central nervous system. It also affects the kidneys and the lungs. Methylmercury, one of the most toxic forms of mercury, is recognized for its detrimental effect on the learning and the neurological development of children.[55]

In the mother, the mercury would eventually cross the placenta. It would accumulate in the liver of the fetus and is set on a protein, the cysteine. Once the child is born, the mercury would accumulate in the kidneys and the brain after leaving the liver.

A pediatrician believes that there is a large number of children with autism among immigrants, because they imposes too many vaccines at the same time upon their arrival in the country. The ratio of the toxicity is another important factor.

The impact of mercury is increasing in a way that "almost exponentially" in the presence of another poison. An experimental test has shown that a dose of infinite mercury that can kill 1 RAT in 100 and a dose of aluminum producing the same effect on the rodent, led to a result entering when combined: no rats in fate unharmed. However, some Vaccines contain aluminum. We can therefore understand better the harmfulness of certain adjuvants for the man.[56]

Therefore, administer at the same time combinations of heavy metals increases their toxicity. According to doctors in Switzerland, all diseases and chronic inflammatory diseases have the heavy metals that lie at the source of the problem.

A double-edged sword

Considering the heavy metals such as neurological toxins, Mercury is found among the most dangerous, because it can cause damage to the central nervous system, disturbances at the level of the neurological function as well as the brain lesions that are therefore sometimes irreversible.

It is impossible to find a study that shows the safety of thimerosal [...]. If you inject this product to an animal, his brain is affected. If you apply on a living tissue, the cell dies. If you insert into a test tube, culture is destroyed. Knowing this, it is impossible to believe that the it can be injected into the body of a baby without causing damage.[57]

The mercury coming from other sources: the contaminated air by heating to coal, the water, the fish, of contraceptive products, shampoos, cosmetics, drops for the eyes, of ointments, makeup removers, mascara, antiseptics, batteries, batteries, lighting, the thermometer, jewelry, dental amalgam, fungicides, germicides, herbicides and insecticides, the paper, the felt, paint, hair lotions, chlorine. The vaccines contain much more mercury than the fruits of the sea.

Forgive them, because they know not what they do!

Some symptoms that we encounter in autistic children are strangely similar to those which have been collected in people who have been poisoned by mercury. There are slurred speech, delays in the development of the language, delays of growth, of motor difficulties, problems of coordination, behavior disorders and

54

hyperactivity. Among other disorders reported include: damage to the nervous system and internal organs, poor perceptions and interpretations, difficulties to manage the information derived from the five senses, of loss of balance, delays in the reflexes physical and mental, of the Emotional irritability, mood, concentration difficulties, difficulties of adaptation, of taste sensitivities that may explain the vagaries food, of sensory defenses, the hypersensitivity to noise and light, the insensitivity to pain explaining the self-mutilation, of personality disorders and a dysfunction of the immune system. Do you not find that there is a great similarity between the symptoms of intoxicated persons to mercury and those of children with autism?

"The exposure to mercury causes immune disorders, sensory, neurological, engines, all similarities generally associated with autism."[58]

The total absence of the language can come from a poisoning in vitro. The mercury would provide behavioral dysfunction, motor, cognitive, neurological, sensory, digestive and immune. It would also amend the immune responses related to food by inhibiting the enzyme functions. It would destroy the neurotransmitters responsible of sleep and emotions. It would prevent the elimination of toxic waste that accumulate in the body thus creating an oxidative stress. It would also affect the functioning of the kidneys and other organs. "Once that mercury is in its intestines, it destroys the intestinal flora, thus favoring the development of microorganisms as the fungus (candida albicans), parasites and bacteria."[59]

Parasitic microorganisms bind to mercury and live there mutually in a form of symbiosis. To eliminate a, it must get rid of the other. The infections will attach where there is heavy metals. Mercury is the last of the toxic elements to leave the body. In addition, it tends to retain the other. The heavy metals, including those from vaccines, help the virus to grab hold of the intestinal wall and the quantity of antibodies that the cover prevents the absorption of nutrients by the villi of the intestinal mucosa.

Many of the disorders classified as psychiatric illness have as origin intoxication to heavy metals. Must it be deduced that all mental illnesses come from a same disorder? God knows how many drugs are sold in psychiatry, whereas a chelation would solve many of the problems.

Nothing goes more

The Mercury must cope with other heads of charge. It was the cause of colitis and ulcers. It night to detoxification in exhausting the amino acids. Several children with autism have a rate of amino acids Low.

Heavy metals can, among other things, inhibit the enzyme activity (including enzymes and coenzymes necessary to the detoxification), produce free radicals and immune disorders, increase the acidity of blood, alter the genetic code, damaging the nervous system, increase allergic reactions, act as antibiotics that can destroy the bacteria both beneficial and pathogens and replace essential minerals in biochemical reactions.[60]

In addition, its antibiotic effect causes a bacterial resistance. It is not recommended to vaccinate a child when he takes of antibiotics and yet of the Vaccines contain or act as such. The prolonged administration of antibiotics would prevent the evacuation of the heavy metals of the system surely because they are attacking the intestinal flora. It must not be vaccinated not more when a child already combat infection, it is apparent or not, which demonstrates the absurdity of multiple injections on a short period of time. Therefore, the Thimerosal also at night to the immunization of virus and bacteria of vaccines. It is contradictory and counter-indicated.

In destabilizing the blood pH, it is the whole body that mercury disrupts. The presence of a bactericidal (mercury) in the intestine is very worrying since the quality of intestinal microbes is necessary to the quality of life. Their loss means a fungal proliferation that destabilizes more the immune system and which poisons the blood system. This explains why the first regression in the autism has place After vaccines and the second, as a result of taking antibiotics.

The lack of Magnesium creates a problem of concentration, the lack of iron cause of the anemia, the deficit in copper leads to problems of digestion and the deficit in calcium provides cardiac anomalies and because of the porosity in the bone density. The presence of heavy metals in our system competes with essential minerals by reducing them. In addition to damage to the nerve cells, mercury is responsible of food allergies in destroying the enzymes related to the degradation of protein molecules, such as that of the gluten, which then act as opiates.

It is also harmful to give a drug against the pain and to bring down the fever after a vaccination. The Fever warns the immune system of a danger. By lowering the fever, the defense system believes that there is no reason to be alarmed. Then, it does not combat during a good time the virus nor the chemical and toxic products of vaccines. These drugs would therefore also have a role to play in the triggering of the autism.

A question of good sense

Mercury has been added to vaccines around 1930. This date corresponds to the first cases identified of autism in children born in the years 1930. The percentage of cases of autism has increased since the beginning of the 1990s after that several vaccines have been added to the calendar and the program. A child is developing normally and autistic becomes after having received one or several vaccines that contain 40 times the dose of heavy metals, which is regarded as unacceptable. It is the obvious.

A mother may have been intoxicated at the mercury if it has been vaccinated being young or during pregnancy. It can therefore transmit a certain amount to her baby despite the placental barriers and thus predispose, especially if it has a weakened immune system or a lazy liver which would render it incapable of well combat all toxins by itself and move them out of his body. If molecules is make up for fabrics encéphaliques of the fetus, neurological problems can ensue. This poor congenital training is often irreversible. The odds are better at a postnatal regression if one wishes to a recovery. This is what makes the difference between be came to the world with autism or be autistic become by regression, or a mixture of the two. The environmental impact of postnatal wake up a sensitivity already acquired before the birth.

(In consulting this site, you will find quotes from several physicians who are opposed to the vaccination: http://www.bickel.fr/128.)

Ignorance, incompetence, negligence, unconsciousness, irresponsibility... or premeditated criminal act?

Between the time of fertilization and before the age of two years, a child may have been exposed to mercury or to one of its derivatives on several occasions, as well as aluminum and formaldehyde, without forgetting the presence of heavy metals in the body of the mother who can reach the fetus. Pregnant women are immunized before, during and after pregnancy. It must also consider all harmful products that pass through the breast milk. Our child has twice received the influenza vaccine to the inside of the same month because a doctor has not checked his book to see if it had been already injected a and was not consulted. This mysterious book of door vaccination a name as ridiculous as "Health Book".

Should he not bear the name of "carnet of new chronic diseases and degenerating"?

Do m bury not alive

Formaldehyde has been used in insulation of homes. It has been regarded as toxic and carcinogenic. Do you remember the scandal surrounding the formaldehyde foam? Prevents that it continues to be used in other construction materials, even after the withdrawal of this foam. I was surprised to see the number of families with a child with autism who live in a newly built house. It is not surprising to consider the increase in the rate of cancer in the population, especially among children, unfortunately. It is also a product used to embalm the dead. The formaldehyde, a known carcinogen, is therefore found in nature in the decaying corpses, which can eventually lead in our groundwater.

Even dentists have used the formaldehyde in the mouth of patients to disinfect the inside of the Teeth; this could explain the cancer of the gums. And yet they claim that it is a harmless substance. If the formaldehyde may develop cancer, can it also be responsible for other types of autoimmune diseases, especially if there is a link between autism, diabetes and cancer?

The GMOS

Genetically modified organisms (GMOS) would be present in the manufacture of some vaccines. In the past, the generic of another drug has been created in genetically modifying a bacterium which produced a soothing substance in order to make this product more efficient than the other. This disturbance has done to ensure that the substance thus created has become toxic and all the people who have used have become paralyzed and with disabilities.

"[...] Of the genetic manipulation that runs poorly escapes to its creators and causes death of men."[61] The victims have not been able to be compensated, because the manufacturing process was protected by a patent, it seems.

The mitochondria and oxidative stress

The survival of living beings depends on their ability to protect themselves against aggression and predators. This are the mitochondria, these parts of the cell that are located between the nucleus and the membrane, which produce the energy necessary for the functioning of cells by converting the nutrients and oxygen. They are therefore responsible for the production of energy in which all bodies need to work well, for as much as there is nothing to impede their work. The brain is one of the bodies that request the most energy. Approximately 20% of children with autism have

58

a mitochondrial dysfunction that translates to the excessive fatigue, of heart and vascular disorder, serious delays of growth and development, the weakness on the plan of the muscle tone and gastrointestinal disorders including constipation, lesions in the brain and diabetes according to the organ affected.

"The U.S. government has recently admitted the vaccinal origin of autistic symptoms of a child with abnormalities of the mitochondria and accepted to this title to compensate the family."[62] Although they claim that it was an isolated case, doctors have demonstrated that there are many cases of malfunction of mitochondria in the autism and that of toxic substances such as environmental thimerosal and the other heavy metals have a fundamental role: they prevent the mitochondria to work well.

Of drugs including those against fever and pain would alter the expression of genes and prevent the production of antioxidants.

This would be one of the reasons for which the vaccines do not make all autistic children, except those who have a genetic predisposition related to a defect of the mitochondria which is increased and accentuated by the presence of heavy metals and other toxins injected or from environmental pollution. Therefore, the vaccines trigger the mitochondrial disease, a pre-existing disorder, which leads to the autism. Spontaneous mutations of the DNA have been found in the blood of the umbilical cord. The mitochondria contain the DNA of the mother. This genetic modification may cause diseases that can become very incapacitating. The risk of disease of course depends on the number of copies of the defective gene or mutation. The attacks can reach the kernel and damage the DNA that will generate by gearing ratio of different cells and outdated. These new cells will be increasingly vulnerable to toxic substances and to the attacks of the environment (air pollution and food). The damage caused to the DNA are often irreparable. Is this that autism will generate a new human race?

"Inadequate disposal of metals, associated with impairment of the antioxidant system of the organism, can thus lead to brain damage due to oxidative stress."[63] The heavy metals would inflate the brain. The increase of its volume has therefore as origin an environmental cause. The ability of detoxification of heavy metals is limited in autistic children. The consumption of antibiotics would decrease the extraction of mercury from approximately 10 per cent. The maturation of the cerebellum is later than that of the rest of the brain, which makes it more vulnerable. The presence of mercury was found in the cerebellum of autistic children and among of the deceased. The oxidative stress in the brain tissue is a marker in people with autism. The oxidative stress causes the death of cells at the origin of neurological lesions postnatal by aggression and by exposure to toxic substances, which affects the cognitive functions, emotions, exploration, to the meaning, to programming and to the traction. The loss of cells leads to the disappearance of the skills and faculties once already acquired such as the language. The loss of cells in the cerebellum is due to attacks and non-developmental anomalies as many would believe.

"A new study supports the thesis according to which the oxidative stress - destruction of cells by of the molecules isolated qualified as free radicals - played a role in the etiology of Autism."[64]

The membrane of our cells leaves return the oxygen and nutrients while preventing bacteria, viruses and toxins to penetrate. Free radicals damage to the cell membrane, which prevents the evacuation of waste and the entry of nutrients. The Oxidative stress can damage the cells by forming a peroxide which is attacking the membrane. This leads to the death of cells.

Oxidative stress is the result of a excessive formation of chemical derivatives unstable, free radicals, even within the cells. In normal conditions, the cell is able to destroy these free radicals. However, in the presence of an excessive accumulation, these molecules are rising to the assault of the cell to stabilize.[65]

In this case, autism would be due to a antioxidant defense disrupted and an increased production of free radicals which have destructive consequences. The oxidation is a form of intoxication. It may well also be a kind of blood poisoning that result. As other signs, there is a rise in the rate of ammonia and acidity in the blood, which disrupts the functioning of blood vessels by a chemical imbalance that can go up to the vascular obstruction by the formation of blood clots. The blood flow thus reduced to the cerebellum led to the death of cells as well as to all the consequences that flow from it. The autistic children suffer from a oxidative stress and abnormalities in the blood stream.

The glutathione, an antioxidant, assistance to immune functions and to the balance gastro-intestinal tract. The heavy metals decrease the antioxidant functions and create a deficit in glutathione. The lack of antioxidants makes the mitochondria more likely to oxidative stress. The treatment by supplements, by enzymes and by oxygen would prove effective in several cases. The food give good defenses against free radicals as green tea, olive oil, onion, garlic and herbs. The antioxidants such as vitamin C désactiveraient free radicals. The minerals essential to tackle also decreasing the oxidative stress, provided that there is enough in the supply of more and more distorted and deficient in essential nutrients, and that the intestines are in fairly good health to absorb and that blood can the route.

After out my son of autism, it remained a disorder of coordination and a deficit of attention which I have remedied by adding supplements that are all connected to deficits of the functioning of the mitochondria. Therefore, attention deficits and the difficulties of learning could be in link with disorders related to the mitochondria. Is it that vaccines are responsible for failures in school?

An opinion

The doctors are not ready to admit that they have committed a crass error, because it was too long ago that they believe in the efficacy and safety of vaccines. It is a little bit like a religious fanatics who do not accept that something else is possible. Confess their wrongs they would lose their credibility and they want to save their reputation and to keep the confidence of the population; they take detours to save time while waiting to find a solution which could The déculpabiliser. They are not on the point not more to accept the Biochemical treatment of autism, since the day where they will accept them, they will at the same time recognize what has caused this pandemic, and this is likely to cost them very expensive in compensation. It would be the same in respect of pharmaceutical companies. It is better to put a dressing on the Bobo to conceal the symptoms.

The voice of a ex-With Autism

My 7 year old son said to me one day: "Mom, I remember when I was with autism. The doctor has done me wrong with a bite on the arm and then I had so badly in the belly that I was no longer able to speak. Later, he gave me another bite and I had even more poorly in the belly and I still had more difficulty to speak. I had evil in the legs and I was no longer able to walk. The feet me chatouillaient and they prevented me from sleeping. This are the doctors who made me sick. I had around 2 years, eh Mom, when it happened?"

As said so well a song: "It has put someone in the world... perhaps it should be the listen.".

Chapter 8

The life inside the intestines

A balance not to break

All systems of the body are affected by the imbalance of the intestinal flora whose immune systems, circulatory, nervous and digestive systems. Each microbe, good or bad, must be at the right place at the right time and in good number to play its role in the health of the individual.

"The Biological correlation of dysfunctions observed in autism almost always start by the processing and by the optimization of the functions of the intestine."[66] The good bacteria such as Lactobacillus and Bifidobactériums (probiotics) reduce the number of harmful bacteria, yeast, molds, fungi and parasites their avoiding to proliferate. After a massive consumption and extended for antibiotics, especially those broad-spectrum, the good bacteria are killed, which allows to fungi and parasites to develop and take the whole place. The balance of our intestinal flora protects us against the diseases, because it stimulates the defense mechanisms.

When living beings draw their nutritive substances in the body of another, such as the inside of his intestines, this can decrease the availability of essential nutrients from the host. Here is what can happen when the balance is broken: by osmosis, the Candida albicans cleans our intestines of organic waste by absorbing their nutrients that are good for him. If it is spreading in large numbers, it changes of form, function, and it becomes a harmful parasite that can penetrate the blood system after having crossed the intestinal membrane. In the blood, it does not feed most of organic waste, but of nutrients essential to the health of the host.

The intestines play a role in the detoxification, digestion, absorption and transport of nutrients as well as in the defenses against infections. It is the central point of our energy. Our belly is the home of our emotions.

Too of hygiene

Who does not know this expression: "too, it is as not enough!" give too much importance to the hygiene can harm and makes it sensitive to allergies of the environment. Before, the children playing in the earth and were continuously in contact with microorganisms. Today, they play on the balconies. They are prohibited from getting dirty when they play outside. They lava and disinfects hands with products more toxic than dirt themselves as soon as they relate to something which awakens our side "paranoid-bugs". Advertisements of Products Household cleaners make us believe that we must fight fiercely and chemically against microorganisms harmless, but supposedly very dangerous.

62

"A house has rarely need to be disinfected; on the contrary, it is of the equilibria stable microbial and protectors that the use of detergent comes compromising, leaving the place to new germs that can even be dangerous."[67] Our body is the home of our intestines.

A territorial struggle

The presence of the Candida, which is a fungus tract, is high among children with autism, especially among those who have received a lot of antibiotics. Approximately 85 per cent of these children have a proliferation in yeasts, viruses, bacteria and other intestinal parasites. The antibiotics would play an important role in the onset of autism: "It was highlighted for many children with autism a presence abnormally high for the yeast which amplifies the behavior problems, concentration and agitation."[68]

The Antibiotics destroy the colonies of beneficial bacteria that make up the intestinal flora natural and combat this fungus. "Anyway, all these pharmaceutical treatments are only trying to camouflage a symptom without ever halt the causative agent."[69] of children have become with autism after having taken too much of antibiotics (and drugs to lower the fever) for repeated ear infections. Among the observed regressions figure the loss of the language. The yeasts promote infections. They can climb up to the throat, the mouth and the nose. Ear infections are caused by bacteria, fungi, parasites and sometimes even by viruses. By destroying the good bacteria of the intestinal flora, antibiotics would weaken and destabilize the immune system, which would aggravate the problem of ear infections repetitive.

This is not just the colon that is irritated

When a intestine is irritated or swollen, it becomes more vulnerable to the presence of unwanted intruders such as bacteria, viruses, parasites and fungi which, adhering to its wall, can the damage. All of these microorganisms, which can cross the intestinal membrane thinned and porous and traveling in the blood and irritate the systems and organs of the body including the brain to impair their optimal functioning. The intestines damaged function poorly, and it follows a bad absorption of nutrients. The Candida albicans affects the uptake and transport of minerals, affects the production of enzymes, prevents the synthesis of vitamins and the metabolism of essential fatty acids: everything the neurotransmitters have need. The brain therefore lack of essential nutrients, since these are the intestines who feed. How can he then well develop and function properly? There is therefore a direct connection, once again between the intestines and the brain. The fatty acids are also necessary for its development and its proper functioning. Unfortunately, a deficiency in this level takes place at the time where the brain in full training in has the most in need.

If food particles are badly digested, they can irritate the intestines more. It is a little as if there was the rake on the membrane. Then, the nutrients may not be absorbed by the blood system from the intestinal villi destroyed and food not degraded. Constipation is a sign of poor digestion and it blocks the absorption of nutrients. The diarrhea, with respect to it, is a way that our body uses to get out of the body and as quickly as possible something that is harmful for him as a food intolerance: too fast for the nutrients are absorbed.

The role of enzymes

The lack of digestive enzymes could be at the origin of the abdominal pain, diarrhea and constipation prolonged, or the alternation of the two. The enzymes decreased Diarrhea and constipation, in addition to destroying the yeasts, but their action is blocked by mercury , lead and aluminum. Minerals are required in the operation of the enzymes, but the heavy metals their compete causing a form of anemia. The vitamins help the enzymes to operate better, provided that they are absorbed and transformed. If the enzymes, including those related to the digestion, are destroyed by heavy metals which inhibit their function, they are no longer able to decompose nor to transform efficiently some foods that trigger allergies and intolerances such as those to gluten and casein.

The pasteurization of milk would destroy enzymes that can help us to degrade the casein and would kill a good part of good bacteria, which would explain the reason for which the previous generations have not experienced problems with dairy products not processed. We should also eat much more of raw foods.

Secretin is a digestive hormone which is also often deficient among people with autism. It improves the language, behavior, stops the diarrhea, gives a better quality of sleep and help with the learning of the cleanliness.

Some enzymes help to the detoxification of the liver overloaded and would also play a role in the regularization of moods. The antioxidant enzymes are disabled by all the waste which come from a porous intestine, which produces a clogging of the system. "A deficiency of the enzyme may therefore have consequences on the operation of the detoxification."[70]

The deficit in enzymes prevents the transformation of a certain amino acid which is essential; it can be transformed and become toxic because it is not metabolized. The accumulation in the body which results can cause a mental retardation. Then, a disability in enzymes can lead to an intellectual disability: another evil in our society which is on the rise. The mechanisms being stuck, the body is no longer able to get rid of waste that accumulate.

"American researchers have announced that they have managed to remove symptoms of mental retardation and autism in rats by inhibiting an enzyme acting on the connections between brain cells, suggesting a possible treatment of these diseases."[71]

The enzymes allow a better communication between neurons, which rule a good part of the hyperactivity, attention deficit, repetitive behaviors and social disabilities.

The nutrient deficit

Processed foods in their preparation lose much of their nutritional values. The same goes for the mode of cooking or of warming used. The genetic modification makes certain nutrients not available. Since the brain is hungry, the Nutritional Deficiency intervenes in the deficit of attention. The hyperactive children have a disability in fatty acids. The delays in the language are related to a deficiency of a nutrient and a bad intestinal absorption.

Intestinal Diseases Chronic prevent the passage of certain vitamins of the family of B vitamins to through the intestinal mucosa, which are essential for the nervous system, which is responsible for some neurological symptoms related to dementia. Intolerance to gluten leads to poor absorption of magnesium, iron and calcium. Children with autism have a deficit in iron and calcium.

Some children with autism in the rich countries are strangely similar to those of the under-developed countries like the children who suffer from malnutrition and famine in Ethiopia who have the distended belly and who are without muscle tone. Approximately 60% of children with autism have gastrointestinal disorders, and they also have the swollen belly as if they were suffering from malnutrition.

We find too much sugar and starch in our current supply, which nourishes the yeasts and other intestinal bacteria effects that love. We consume too many sugary foods because we lack of energy, although that produced by the sugars to be false and acts that on a short duration. In addition, caffeine irritates the intestines. The more one takes, the more it is tired and more we need it, because the coffee would prevent the absorption of iron, which makes us even more tired. This dependence creates a vicious circle.

It is therefore obvious to consider autism as a physical illness which disrupts the brain rather than as a mental disability irreversible. It is a bad functioning of the digestive systems and tract leads to a immune disorder, and Neurological which is reflected by strange behaviors. It is a nutrient deficit accompanied by a general intoxication.

Wicked small bugs

The yeasts may be transmitted to the child by the mother if she has been affected during her pregnancy or birth. Normally, the proliferation of this fungus comes of uses repeated and prolonged for contraceptives and antibiotics, contacts with heavy metals and chemicals such as pesticides; it is encouraged by a bad diet rich in sugar and flour. The yeasts also like dairy products and an environment acid. It must also avoid acid fruits because they love them. It should therefore not feed them with what they love. The infant milk formula would contribute to the yeasts. Streptococcus transmitted from the mother to the child would be at the origin of the nervous tics.

Some yeasts may emanate of toxins in the form of miasmas (gas) which cross the intestinal membrane and create a form of intoxication to toxic fumes. It is as if the child had gas in the neurons. The yeasts also produce a form of acid thus modifying the blood pH, which influence the circulatory system. The toxic fumes depleted again the immune system. The candida product of waste which affect the nervous and circulatory systems. It would therefore be a blood poisoning progressive.

"The brain can be affected by the toxins of the Candida, thus causing loss of memory, changes in mood and concentration difficulties."[72] depression, frustration, irritability and anxiety are also part of it. Since there is a direct relationship between the brain and the intestine, the brain is affected by the toxic environment intestinal tract. The toxins produced interfere in the functions of the brain and the Intestinal, therefore also immune.

"The yeasts genetically transform certain human cells that surround the digestive tract. Certain human cells, therefore, may contain the DNA own to the yeasts."[73] Of analyzes reveal the presence of yeasts in the blood and urine. The aggressiveness, behavioral disorders and hyperactivity could well be signs of the presence of intestinal parasites. The fact that a child grinding of teeth at night would be a good indication also.

To defeat the yeasts, it must avoid certain foods (sweetened, floury, acids), chemicals, drugs and other medical treatments such as the anesthesias, balancing the whole with the addition of multivitamins and minerals, the essential fats such as oils Omega, enzymes, antioxidants and probiotics. The antifungal treatments reduce the hyperactivity, improve the visual contact, the language, the sleep and the concentration.

After the yeast come in second order the intestinal bacteria. The substances released by these parasites speakers with the substances that we produce and which are necessary for the proper functioning of the thyroid gland and the neurological functions. Their Toxins interfere with the chemistry of the brain. These toxins injected into the brain of rats during experiments have given them the behaviors that are similar to those of autism. The toxins which accumulate may have an effect on the Microbial imbalance that they increase, can influence the digestion and absorption of nutrients, intestinal permeability as well as the immune functions.

And this is also the case concerning the bacterium Clostridium. "The emergence of yeasts and bacteria of type Clostridium develops as a result of the administration of long doses of antibiotics."[74]

It ends by Y develop a resistance and the same applies to the antibiotics that are found in our food chain from treated animals and whose we consume the flesh. The flesh of the animals treated with antibiotics destroyed the intestinal flora of those who feed on it. That is why the intensive livestock production contributes in some way to the emergence of the autism.

The nutrient deficiency helps the Clostridium to grow and expand by immune deficiency. The yeasts can transform the sugars (and carbohydrates) Phenol, a substance close to the alcohol, which creates among persons with autism a sensation and a behavior which are akin to a form of drunkenness. Barley, wheat, grapes and apples are used in the production of alcoholic products. It is therefore necessary to avoid foods that can ferment, especially in the case of infections to the yeasts. Remove the skin of these fruits can decrease the intestinal fermentation.

Take out the trash

To our death, yeasts as enzymes and other pests such as worms help our body to decompose. Our Intestines work as a treatment plant, purification and filtration of contents ingurgitées, but in the case of incorrect operation, they become a dump where accumulate waste that rot and emit fumes.

We eat too much meat and not enough fruits and vegetables (fiber). If we reduce our consumption of meat, we could save the planet, since too large a quantity of cereals are used to feed the animals for slaughter, then they could feed the inhabitants of the regions under-fed.

Let us go back to the bacterial growth. There are toxic fumes that emerge of waste rotten. When diarrhea or constipation or alternating, the elimination and absorption are wrong. Diarrhea very smelly can come from the decay of the crust of rotten meat that is glued to the inside of the intestines, and sometimes, this are liquids which are coming out of a plug of constipation. The putrefaction of the stool product of the ammonia and the gas. The Ammonia, which goes to the blood by intestinal porosity also travels to the brain. It is as if the child had the blood poisoned. The toxic substances produced by fermentation and putrefaction lead to intoxication. The accumulation of waste reactions in the body destroyed the health in general.

The Die Off

The use of noise and probiotics can help to restore order in the intestinal flora. In several cases, it must also appeal to an antiviral to completely get rid of viruses from the vaccinations. It must be certain that the parasites have not developed of insensitivity to the treatments.

In addition, he must expect to a strong reaction that is called die off. During this period, the child may have an increase of autistic behaviors, because the yeasts, dying, deflate and emptied of their toxins. The use of activated charcoal absorbs these toxins, but also all the nutrients. Therefore, it must be careful. This strong reaction demonstrates once again that there is a link between the intestines and the brain.

The biofilm

The yeasts prevent the heavy metals out, and vice versa. The bacteria, microbes, the parasites and the yeasts may manufacture their biofilm (a protective membrane to prevent the immune system to achieve) using the heavy metals such as mercury. They also use our minerals such as iron, making them non-available to our organization. "The Biofilms are a Matrix gelatinous () secreted by bacteria opportunists and yeast. These pathogens secrete these biofilms as a defense mechanism to avoid any immune detection that allows them to survive in an environment hostile otherwise."[75]

Even antibiotics and probiotics do not arrive to join. Of specific enzymes, often deficient among persons with autism, expose the yeasts and bacteria harmful to other attacks in breaking the screen protector. It must fight simultaneously and alternately to the time against the yeasts, parasites and heavy metals.

The fluorine, accomplice of heavy metals

"The metabolic ions (heavy metals) are absorbed by the wall (intestinal), and then react with certain membrane enzymes by destroying them."[76] The mercury and cadmium degrade the intestinal mucosa, which would result in a microbial proliferation and a high production of neurotoxins. The intestinal mucosa is sensitive to oxidative stress. The heavy metals play an important role in the oxidation. Weakening the intestinal membrane, the Heavy Metals The make them also porous, and are therefore responsible for the consequences. Vaccines, antibiotics and contraceptives would contribute to the decline of the impermeability of the bowel, which amends the functions of our defense mechanism.

If the aluminum fluoride exists, there could therefore be of aluminum in the toothpaste. In addition, fluorine would increase the absorption of aluminum by our Organization. It abîmerait the enamel of the teeth because it would destroy the enzymes that form, which would give more work to the dentists. Hard to believe, is it not? It would also affect the enzymes related to the prédigestion and digestion. The fluoridation of water would be responsible for dental caries and digestive disorders.

"Fluorine interferes with the metabolism of calcium and phosphorus as well as on the functioning of the glands parathyroid and enzymes."[77] It would be a thyroid disruptive and a factor mutagenic. Its toxic substance would be dangerous to human health, because it would accumulate in the body where the latter is unable to evacuate. Here is the dictionary definition for the word "fluorine": "Gas greenish yellow very dangerous to breathe." A intoxication in fluorine would result of neurological disorders. It is difficult to ask the children not to swallow toothpaste. Even after being well rinsed the mouth, traces remain. Fluorine would be a poison for the OS and the nervous system.

The level of fluoride in the blood is increasing steadily as a result of the prolonged use of fluoridated toothpaste. Fluorine crosses the blood-brain barrier, producing biochemical disorders functional

69

and at the level of the nervous system during the development period of infancy and childhood [...]. The enzymes present in raw foods are indispensable to their own digestion [...] fluorine destroyed much of enzymes [...]. The scientists of the University of San Diego have also demonstrated that the fluorine mutait out of service a specific enzyme of the body responsible for the transport of oxygen breathing. It destroys the hemoglobin, creating severe anemia. It would be a determining factor in the decline of the intellectual quotient observed in several countries where the fluoridation of water is systematic.[78]

The Sun and the Vitamin D

Vitamin D is essential for the proper functioning of the brain and intestines, which has just confirm once more a link between these two parts of the body.

The rays of the sun are essential to our survival. We need to maintain in Health The immune system, to metabolize properly our nutrients, to facilitate the production of certain nutrients, including vitamin D. our skin and our eyes need to receive the light of the sun, with the entire spectrum and without restrictions [...] to maintain our health at a minimum, one hour per day.[79]

The vitamin D deficiency disrupts the immune response, deteriorates the physical faculties and the brain and participates in the development of the Celiac disease (gluten intolerance). The lack of this essential vitamin contributes to the development of autoimmune diseases and fact decline the cognitive faculties. It therefore plays a role in the intellectual performance.

"The autism was more frequent in the regions where the UVB radiation was lower as the towns in areas with significant air pollution or those who had frequent rain."[80]

The female hormones and masculine have different effects on the production and the assimilation of vitamin D. This last is important for the development and the functioning of the brain. A lack of this vitamin fact swell the brain, thus increasing its surface area, which can also create an atrophy of the brain and brain damage. "The apparent increase in the prevalence of autism in the course of the last 20 years corresponds to the increase of medical advice to avoid the sun, the councils which have reduced the levels of vitamin D."[81] The vitamin D plays a role in the maintenance of the sealing of the intestinal barrier at the level of the integrity of tight junctions of the mucosa.

The stool

Since that the stool of our son are normal, it seems to be less susceptible to infections, which proves that the intestines have a direct link with the immune system. When he catches a cold, it the combat more easily and more quickly. Therefore, intestinal health could have an impact on the defense mechanisms.

One evening, in returning to the day care center, our son had very badly in the stomach. Sitting on the sofa, he was to make the larger "flapping" of hands never seen, by shaking the head The eyes turned toward the ceiling. It also gave blows to the head against the folder. It was more of a year that he no longer had presented these symptoms. When the next morning, I realized that he was suffering from a gastroenteritis, I understood up to what point an intestinal disorder may cause a neurological imbalance which is characterized by a strange behavior as the autistic symptoms. I have no more doubt about it: autism is not a mental illness incurable. It is intestinal disease which is trafficking. Since this is the case, it would mean that the intestinal diseases could also be the cause of various psychiatric illnesses.

Chapter 9

The allergies, intolerances and sensitivities of food

The Behavioral Reactions

There has food allergies say hidden. They are difficult to soupçonnables, because they do not cause spontaneous reactions as violent as those we know under the name of anaphylactic shock. There is therefore the reactions in the medium and long terms which appear only a few hours or days after the consumption of the food concerned, which can modify the behavior.

If the allergy is the tip of the iceberg and the submerged part would represent the intolerances; and it is what is not seen to cause problems.

A German doctor, Joseph Egger, has been one of the pioneers to make the link between allergies and mental health [...]. The results have shown that the allergenic foods alone were capable of causing severe depressions, nervousness, feelings of anger without object, a lack of motivation and absences severe mental. The foods that have caused the most reactions were wheat, milk, sugar and eggs. The inflammatory state caused by the allergic reaction in all these cases ranging from depression to autism is probably one of the main mechanisms by which the food allergy affects the brain.[82]

The physical and psychological problems may be related to allergies say "the brain". Here is the story of a small boy who was told to me by an occupational therapist: "A boy who had of autistic symptoms suffered from acute constipation and prolonged. It was remained nine days and more without being able to evacuate its stools. During his hospitalization, which lasted approximately three weeks, if I remember well, it has been fed by intravenous users. To the great surprise of the parents when they came to the visit, he started to talk about, to smile and to have a visual contact.

"Once healed, he returns to the House and start eating again as before. It is regressing and its autistic symptoms resurface. The parents then have understood that the power supply has a role to play. After having followed a diet without gluten or casein and by removing other food allergens, its stool are become beautiful and it is set to act as a normal child." This are therefore of intolerance or food allergies which would create a bad intestinal operation causing neurological disorders. If the intestines work well, the brain will be better for it.

Allergies do not always occur by breathing difficulties or by skin irritation, but they assert themselves by other physical or psychological problems take time to appear. And this can go for two to three days later, which makes it difficult for the establishment of a link of cause and effect. A abnormal behavior would come from a biochemical disorder. An autoimmune disease resembles an allergy toward his own body.

The Immune disorders

Of immune disorders may have an effect on the brain tissue and nervous. The similarity of functions between the cells of the immune system and those of the central nervous system takes a same origin during the embryonic stage. They play a similar role in the perception of the environment. One develops a memory cognitive called while the other develops an immune memory. This indicates, once more, a link between the immune system and the brain.

A disorder in the home of one of them may cause simultaneously a disorder in the other. When the immune system reacts too strongly, this gives the impact on the central nervous system. In what way? If an immune response is too strong, it can, by inflammation, cause lesions of the intestines as well as the brain. It could therefore establish a link between these lesions and the Intestinal porosity as that of myelin. "A study published in the Acta Paediatrica confirms that 43% of children with autism have the intestinal mucosa permeable."[83]

The allergies, just as the food intolerances, occur when the immune system reacts too strongly against a food that it treats it as an

72

invader enemy. The same applies to the infections. Me, for example , I have an immune system overthrown. The antibodies that I should have in greater quantity are those that I have in more small number, and those that I have the least are those that I should have the most, which fact that I react too strongly and inadequately to an infection. It is an imbalance between the Th1 and Th2. This would explain the increase of cancer and autoimmune diseases in the population (diabetes, autism, celiac disease). Allergies are also in full expansion. The immune system is reversed and out of adjustment.

I therefore what is called an autoimmune disease. This demonstrates why my son has had a adverse reaction to vaccines that have led to the development of autism. If the doctors took the time to check the field and the Medical history Family, many tragic accidents could have been avoided in the past and several may be in the future also.

A deficit in IgA antibodies would be caused by frequent infections vaccine () Bacterial, viral and parasitic diseases. Too many provocations destabilize the antibodies and overthrew the immune system. Our Organization has become too sensitive to environmental attacks multiple. Reduce the stress on the immune system decreases behavioral disorders and delays in development.

A defective plumbing

It is thanks to the intestines If the nutrients needed for the operation of all the Organization are absorbed and distributed where the need is felt. On the other hand, they also prevent the penetration of toxic components and microorganisms in our body. The intestinal mucosa is a barrier that protects our interior of the outside world.

"A normal colon and healthy today is an endangered species. There is simply more [...] the only place where you can still see a normal colon today is in your book of anatomy."[84]

Gastrointestinal disorders affected more than 20 per cent of the population there is about 10 years, and we are talking here only of persons who have been diagnosed. How many people are unaware that their physical or mental health problems may find their origins in the intestinal functions?

When the mucosa is permeable (as a mosquito net with large holes), it can let go of undesirable elements as of undigested proteins , bacteria, fungi and heavy metals [...]. If undigested proteins enter the bloodstream, an immune reaction occurs.[85]

Among all the foreign substances traveling in the body after having crossed the intestinal mucosa porous, defense mechanisms may have difficulty to distinguish between what is dangerous and what is not because there is too much of toxins and strange materials present at the same time.

The irritation and inflammation of the intestinal mucosa gives rise to what is called the syndrome of the intestine porous and to the release of large food proteins in the circulation. For the immune system, these proteins represent toxins. Their presence causes an immune reaction which is manifested clinically by food allergies. Among persons with autism, food allergies come increase problems immunity already present. In addition, food allergens exacerbate gastrointestinal disorders and can often exacerbate the problems of behavior exhibited by a child.[86]

The Allergies, ignored and not processed on time would result in other food allergies. The particles of food and protein badly digested which are found in the blood system are at the origin of the outbreak of allergies related to the power supply. After having passed through the intestinal mucosa, they have requested the immune system to produce antibodies against these foods. This is not normal that a child of 4 years has 21 allergies and 40 food intolerances on 93 foods tested! Is it normal to produce as much antibody against the food we consume?

All antibodies which adhere to the intestinal wall can irritate even more while increasing its porosity. If the intestinal mucosa becomes more and more thin and porous, it therefore leaves pass more large quantities of harmful substances and food particles badly digested in the blood and lymphatic systems that trigger other immune responses producing other antibodies which still adhere to the intestinal wall, and the problem is getting worse. This would be in this way that other food allergies can be created from the first. The best way to solve this problem is to eliminate all food allergens. A decline of antibodies in the blood decreases at the same time the symptoms and allows a better flow of oxygen and nutrients to the cells that remained in lack.

"Mothers of children with autism have noticed that the making of certain allergenic foods coincides with the increase of the autistic behaviors."[87] Approximately 81 per cent of children improve with the elimination of the gluten and casein. Food opioids inhibit the receptors and neurotransmitters in acting on the GABA, which causes the stereotyped behaviors. The gluten allergies and casein give of neurological disorders chronic sometimes.

The Opioids

It is a drug strong causing a dependency almost as severe as heroin. If the weakening of the immune system has created a intestinal permeability, these peptides of opioids spend in the bloodstream causing a dependency (such as drugs), affecting the neurological transmission and can induce behavioral difficulties and regressions of language as seen in autism. The persons suffering from such food allergies brain say often have a pronounced taste for the food that they do not tolerate. This is because a first bite gives them the impression of improving a depressive state or even a sense of euphoria and well-being. The process becomes, subsequently, more toxic than allergen. The results are related to a poisoning rather than to an extreme sensitivity, but at the base, there is an immunity totally deficient and intestinal disease.[88]

Intestinal inflammation can be caused by heavy metals, vaccines, antibiotics, viruses, bacteria, a zinc deficiency, Immune Disorders and intolerance to gluten and casein. Mercury binds to the intestinal mucosa in the irritant. When the inflammation is manifest, it is as if a part of the intestine is inflating like a balloon. By this very fact, the mucosa becomes thinner with more space between the cells. "More and more data to suggest that some vaccines could play a role on the gastrointestinal inflammation which usually suffer autistic children (Wakefield). In addition, components of several vaccines may cause autoimmune reactions."[89]

The difficulty digesting dairy products could well come from a viral infection and vaccination. Gastrointestinal disorders lead to food intolerances and allergies cause gastro-intestinal disorders. It is another vicious circle.

Although there seems to be turning in a circle, it is that the human body is as an engine to Workings: when a mechanism is blocked, this causes repercussions elsewhere; this is why it is necessary to consider the holistic approach of the human body.

The intestinal permeability can also be caused by antibiotics, yeasts, alcohol, certain drugs against fever and pain, infections, simultaneous multiple and the stress of the immune system. That is why we need to avoid giving a drug against the fever to a child whose life is not necessarily in danger to the risk that it develops a intestinal porosity with food allergies arising therefrom.

The proteins partially digested (gluten, casein, soybean) can irritate the complex structure of endomorphins that the nervous system uses to calm the pain, which would explain why some children with autism self injure because of an insensitivity to pain while other are hypersensitive to sound and light. Opiates bind on the molecules of the receptors causing poor eye contact and language difficulties. That is why the withdrawal of the casein and soy has enabled many children to unlock on the plan of the verbal communication. The reaction to certain foods causes an aggressive behavior and sometimes even this can go up to convulsions. The opioids of peptides are as of the morphine which is sabotaging the neurotransmitters.

Some products causes of allergies can interfere with each other. In other words, the consumption of a food alone will not cause any reaction, but the consumption of two products causes of allergies mild or moderate at the same time can stimulate an allergic response by excessive load in the system.[90]

The combination of two or several allergenic foods accentuates the reaction. This is where the food combinations are taken into account. And this allergic load often comes from a too large intestinal porosity. The most common allergy are those to peanut, nuts, eggs, shellfish, fish, milk, soy, wheat, etc. Now, we can add the sesame to the list.

As a result of the presence of these heavy metals, the normal assimilation of food is restricted and transforms those in toxins which will be stored by the body. These toxins, opioids, migrate up to the receptors in the brain and can be the cause of psychiatric illness serious such as autism, schizophrenia, hyperactivity, depression [...]. Finally, the ancestor of the wheat, the grand spelt, had 7 pairs of chromosomes. Since then, the small spelt appeared in the Middle Ages into account 21 pairs as the current wheats. However, the human being does not have the ability to digest of the wheats comprising more than 7 pairs of chromosomes.[91]

What have we done to wheat for the have transformed into poison too sneaky since the industrial era? Eczema and other skin diseases would be signs of food intolerances, but of course, the pharmaceutical companies love the income facts with the creams prescribed. Those who suffer from irritable bowel syndrome should refrain from eating eggs, because the albumin of the egg would prevent the colon to repair. Celiac Disease, Crohn's disease and colitis to ulcers would affect a person on four. Several doctors are unaware of the link between certain diseases and food allergies. Then, they go back to the school in training continues!!!

Since a few years, there has been a resurgence of unprecedented intolerances in gluten, which means that we no longer have enough enzymes to digest completely or not of enzymes of everything. A large protein that is not digested in full in our small intestine by lack of enzymes creates very serious health problems. Currently, the medicine is not dealing with it. The small intestine is a body ignored by the medical corps. But it represents the center of the body.[92]

The casein and gluten would have become real poisons to some people. The feed could therefore be a factor of intoxication. For example, if we give the chocolate to a dog, it may die because it cannot digest. It can therefore be poison gradually with the food that we cannot digest or assimilate, either because it was not the enzymes that it takes to their degradation or simply because our system is not done to receive this kind of power, without forgetting all the chemicals that accompany it and who are also hurt our intestines.

In the perspective of the general intolerance to milk cow and the food security, mention should be made of the possible presence of contaminants: hormones, antibiotics, pesticides, dioxins. Sanitary controls should allow to delete such contamination that can only undermine the biological functions and to the health of the consumer.[93]

It would be the consequences resulting from the mégaproduction Agri-Food. The lactose and casein from goat milk would be more easy to digest and to tolerate for people the less sensitive. It would be the same concerning the milk of from other than that of Holstein cows. By desire to increase the production and at the same time revenues, the farmers would have the wrong breed of cattle dairy. The swellings, flatulence and gases are signs of lactose intolerance to same that the abdominal pain, diarrhea, nausea and dehydration. These morphines will by the blood, anywhere in the body. They are the basis of degenerating diseases and rheumatism. How to attack? First, it depends on our genetic heritage; then, if the witness is fragile on the psychic plane, this will be the depression or insomnia that will install or disorders of learning and concentration; if the field is allergic, intolerances will surface; if it is a Muscle weakness, rheumatism and arthritis will take place; but if the brain is immature, this are autistic traits that will appear.

The biological evidence. The pervasive developmental disorders caused by the partial degradation of the gluten and casein have been highlighted in several medical publications written in particular by Professor Reichelt of the Institute of paediatric research of the University of aslo. The Biochemical disorder facing

77

the body during an intoxication to gluten and casein is at the origin of a wide range of behavioral disorders ranging from hyperactivity to autism in passing by the personality disorders and epilepsy.[94]

The field of epilepsy would disrupt the language that can be also due to a lack of vitamin B6. The Biochemical treatments give better results than the drug treatments on this subject, because they do not just camouflage evil, but they resolve the cause.

A review to the Magnifying Glass

The results of the tests and blood tests to detect food allergies in Canada in hospitals do not disclose any, because they are not as sensitive as those who are made elsewhere in specialized laboratories in the pervasive developmental disorders in the United States, and some but very little in Europe. It takes a certain percentage of antibodies for that the process used to capture and thereby give a positive result. Why the test done in Quebec revealed-it only two allergies in our son: the beef protein and peanuts, whereas the test done in the United States demonstrated 10 allergies serious to moderate which a severe sesame seeds, without forgetting its many intolerances and sensitivities categorized among the allergies medium to light? Despite his allergy marked to bovine protein, a pediatrician to a hospital for children in a specialized clinic in power in Montreal we stated that we could continue to give dairy products to our son. Fortunately, we did not follow its recommendations because the result of the tests of food analyzes made with the LPG (Great Plains Laboratory, Kansas) revealed that he is allergic to all dairy products, between other casein.

Skin tests do not cover any since they would appeal to a certain type of antibody which reactions are in the short term, whereas in the case of autism, this are antibodies which reactions are in the long term that are associated with behavior disorders. There is allergic reactions to delaying: sleep disorder, bad urinary control, sinusitis, otitis, irritation, etc.

The IgE antibodies would be responsible for the immediate allergic reactions including those that cause inflammation. They make the parasites inactive, monitor the cancerous cells and cause the anaphylactic shock. IgM give the first attack against a new infection, whereas the IgG give the resistance to the body against a infection already view. The IgA protect the intestines and the digestive tube against the microorganisms. They would be secreted by the gallbladder when it works well and that it has not been withdrawn because of calculations. The IgA determine the celiac disease and because they are sometimes the antibodies the least abundant in the blood Normally, the results of the analyzes are often negative. "These tests may produce false negative results. For example, the results of the tests IgA, EMA and TTg will be falsely negative among individuals who have a deficiency of IgA, which occurs in 3 % of patients with celiac disease."[95]

Concerning the screening of the celiac disease, it must check before the test if the person has a deficit in IgA to avoid potential false negative results. Doctors and parents rely too much to these results for decide to initiate the diet or not.

A biopsy would give better results, as long as it is practiced in the proper place. It also has its limits since it can be intolerant to gluten in presenting little intestinal atrophies. At the beginning of the disease, the atrophy of the villi may be too slight to highlight the diagnosis. In addition, the severity of the lesions may vary from one place to another.

Only a third of patients with neurological disorders associated with the sensitivity to gluten has a villous atrophy during a duodenal biopsy. Even some patients with biochemical markers of malabsorption (since the villi reduced prevent the absorption of nutrients) as a serological rate bottom of vitamin B12, folic acid or vitamin D had a duodenal histology normal. These cases can illustrate the uneven nature of the participation of the intestine in celiac disease and the interpretation imprecise of duodenal biopsies by the histo-pathologists inexperienced. Preliminary data based on the count of the sub-population of T cell in the epithelium of the small intestine suggest that these patients have a celiac disease potential. There are however of patients where the immunological disorder is mainly directed to the nervous system with little or no damage at the level of the intestine.[96]

The best tests remain the withdrawal of the allergenic food concerned follow-up of observations concerning the improvement or the disappearance of the symptoms that are related. And then, to restore the food and note the changes. It is the best way.

Ramonons The Fireplace

Several chronic diseases are in relationship with our food, our intestinal flora and our digestive system. The bread and pastries to basis of gluten, same as the melted cheese stick to the dishes. They also adhere to the same way to the wall of our intestines and even more when they are combined. The modification of the protein of wheat through the centuries has made even more sticky. Our Intestines clog up a toxic layer which adheres to its Wall and the intestine is no longer able to get rid of it. The organization becomes oversaturated. Then, the foods not degraded fermenting and putréfient resulting in an imbalance of the intestinal ecosystem.

The putrefaction of protein product of the ammonia and of phenol, of toxic substances. The stool too dry from the constipation destroy the lactobacilli which constitute the intestinal flora, which leaves more to the microbes of putrefaction. The corpses of bacteria y would also contribute.

A bad functioning of the intestines can lead to cancer. The intestine has 24 hours to eliminate the waste from the power supply. If it is not working properly, deposits of waste accumulate on its wall, which can damage the villi and prevent the absorption of nutrients. These deposits of faeces can reach several centimeters thick and have a consistency of a tire! These wastes can in the long run prevent the absorption and the penetration in the body of the vitamins and mineral salts. The chronic bowel disorders can thus be at the origin of a nutritional deficiency, regardless of the amount of food or the quantity of vitamins absorbed.[97]

The stagnation of contents creates a chronic irritation to the intestinal walls which leads to another form of inflammation, which aggravates the nutrient deficiencies, and the brain is as well hungry and thirsty.

Processed foods to basis of refined flour and sugar are difficult to digest and poorly nutritious. Our modern diet is inadequate and it flies in the face of our genetic heritage from the Paleolithic period where our ancestors hunted, fished and gathered to feed. Then, agriculture and livestock have emerged with the sedentary lifestyle.

"It differs from the food that he considers as potentially harmful to the human body: the food cooked at high temperature and also, among other things, wheat and dairy products, and favors organic food."[98] It should return to a ancestral nutrition, original, regional and natural.

The indoor pollution

The fermentation and putrefaction in the interior of the intestine alter the intestinal flora of a considerable way. Normal stool have almost no smell. Let us return in the following context.

This possibility stems from the absence of enzymes capable of "cut" the giant proteins (lactoglobulin; gliadin) [...]. These lead putréfactions a state of local inflammation and general, predisposing for triggering or to the worsening of autoimmune diseases (polyarthritis, acute episodes of neurological disorders),

Allergies Lung or the epidermal cells, without forgetting the intestinal problems evident (bloating, gas, hemorrhagic colitis).[99] The production of lactase, an enzyme to digest the lactose, which is a natural sugar found in milk, ceases after the age of two years. This are the enzymes which allow to cut food so that they can be assimilated by our Organization. The Europeans and North Americans are those who have the least. Those who can digest the milk to the adult age would be extremely unlikely to a mutation abnormal due to environmental impacts or by some form of natural selection. When the intestinal microorganisms ferment lactose, it is the result of abundant gas and flatulence. When the intestines are porous, these gases are traveling in the blood and make it to the brain where they can cause emotional disorders such as mood swings or aggressive behavior.

Under the influence of various factors: genetic (enzyme deficiency, predisposing field, allergies) and environmental as the modern diet (including the gluten, the proteins of the milk and milk products of cooking to high temperature) or the frequent socket of chemical substances such as antibiotics, the intestinal mucosa would be attacked, weakened and made too permeable thus facilitating the passage in the blood circulation of bacterial macromolecules and food. The residues in food or bacterial would be captured by the immune system, and then directed to the natural émonctoires causing inflammation of the target organ.[100]

The toxins are pick up a little everywhere in the body and attack to the place the more sensitive of the body. The intolerance and the lack of enzymes transform the proteins in toxic substances. The accumulation creates a gradual poisoning, cause inflammation and difficulties in functioning in various parts of the body. For example, arthritis is an accumulation of waste in the joints, causing their degeneration. The accumulation of material acidifies the field and destroys the cells.

The excess toxins from the intestinal permeability overload the liver which produces less of enzymes and bile, making the digestion even less effective.

The accumulation of toxins may have an effect on immune function, intestinal permeability, digestion and assimilation of nutrients and it further increases the microbial imbalance. The inflammation due to microbial infections, to food allergies, to toxins endogenous and exogenous, as well as a nutritional state sub-optimal make the fabric gastro-intestinal tract less resistant to oxidative stress. We must not lose sight of the fact that the self-gastrointestinal immunity could be one of the causes of the chronic bowel inflammation, particularly when there is the presence of heavy metals which plays an important role on the plan of the oxidation.[101]

The presence of heavy metals increased the rate of antibodies. In addition, the chronic bowel inflammation creates a oxidative stress on the mucosa, which fact decrease the production of enzymes secreted by the intestinal villi. This oxidative stress is caused by microbial proliferation , the nutrient deficiency, a bad digestion and the taking of antibiotics that alter the intestinal flora.

These food intolerances can be caused by pollution in the small intestine of microbial genera [...] the inadequacy of pancreatic secretion and bile, a bad power supply, but also the intoxication to heavy metals. Heavy metals are secure on the enzymes and block their action in the entire organization. They have an inhibitory action on the peptidases intended for the digestion of the gluten and casein. These proteins badly digested spend in the blood system in the form of opiate peptides and attach to the receptors in the brain, which may cause degeneration in the body.[102]

Food can act as of hard drugs, because they induiraient among people sensitive substances close to those recognized and used in pharmacology as histamine and serotonin.

Intestinal parasites also ferment carbohydrates and produce it in the alcohol which would alter the structure of proteins that are responsible for autoimmune reactions; that is why some children with autism must follow a specific diet. They produce toxins which are overloading the liver even more, which pollutes the blood more and poisons all cells of the body.

The bacterium Clostridia inhibits the growth and mental functions of the child. Of bad bacteria transform sulphates which are essential for the detoxification and for the proper functioning of the neurotransmitters in sulphites toxic. That is why a doctor believes in the improvement of certain stereotypes linked to autism by the use of a specific antibiotic to these bacteria. It must, however, make attention with antibiotics for not further damage the intestinal flora already if weakened with those broad-spectrum. I would not be surprised that we propose soon a vaccine against autism, but it will at that time be on our guard and prudence.

"The most serious consequence is without doubt the toxic poisoning linked to the development of pathogenic germs. It occurs a true self-intoxication."[103] A combination of toxins makes it even more toxic. It should be well hydrated to allow for the evacuation. Tea, coffee and alcohol contribute to dehydration of the body, slows down the digestion and gives of stress in the liver. We do not drink enough water is alkaline.

Our charge batteries

The enzymes are the source of our energy. "Enzymes are the substances which are that life is possible. They are essential to each of the chemical reactions that occur in the body. Without enzymes, there would be no activity."[104]

Our cells need to be well fed to keep us in good health and enzymes are important to transform our food and route the nutrients to cells. In addition to assisting the nutrients to be properly assimilated, enzymes support the immune system in its task.

"The enzymes involved in the times on our ability to capture the energy of food and to regenerate our body. An imbalance of our resources in enzymes leads inevitably to a degeneration and to a decline in the immune system."[105]

The enzymes trigger certain chemical reactions in the body. They break down proteins into amino acids. If the other components that are involved in this transformation are present and effective. They react to a protein or a food additive. Of the enzymes improve digestion and the absorption of nutrients. This is found in the saliva, the stomach, pancreas and intestines. If you eat too fast, there digests less well, because there was not enough mastiqué for that the enzymes of the saliva begin the digestion. When the pancreas suffers from a lack of enzymes, it swells to counter the request and to respond to the work required. The Fever produces enzymes to combat a bacterial infection. Prevent the fever to do its job leaves the infection is Establish and advance.

If the body has less need to secrete digestive enzymes to respond to the request, it can no longer take care of the operation of the metabolism on the plans of the energy and the cellular detoxification. They also have the role of a catalyst in some recombinant molecules. Each type of enzymes has a specific function and can change of function to the need. If it is necessary for the body to produce more of digestive enzymes, this makes the metabolic enzymes less available for the functions of the immune system, because the metabolic enzymes to leave their work to go and help the digestive enzymes; then, the Cellular cleaning is not done during this time. Among the two types of enzymes, those related to metabolism are involved in the training, the repair and operation of all the cells of the body; whereas those digestive say are involved in the decomposition of fat, protein and carbohydrates. When the metabolic enzymes must come to the aid of the digestive enzymes, it results in less available energy to cells and more of the toxins in circulation.

"The glands and most of the organs, including the brain, suffer enormously from this disability. The latter can in effect be atrophy due to a power supply essentially composed of processed products devoid of these enzymes in which the organization has so desperately need."[106] The lack of enzymes is an important factor in the onset of food allergies. It is also responsible for swelling, gas and of heartburn. The enzymes fractionate the large molecules into smaller so that they can be more easily assimilated.

Processed foods by the agri-food industry cause the occurrence of chronic diseases. The causes of our current deficit in enzymes are located in the food treatments such as cooking and processing and storage. All be living plant or animal contains enzymes that contribute to their own organic deterioration when they die, which is the same when the plants or animals are consumed: their enzymes help to their digestion.

"Once they have reached the small intestine, these substances (mercury) can bind and disable of the enzymes necessary for digestion."[107] Among the other enemies of enzymes are located: free radicals, some radiation, chemotherapy, as well as of food particles and bacteria which originate from a porous intestine. But the mercury would be one of their worst enemies, because it amends the immune response, inactive enzymes related to the digestion of proteins opioids and creates deficiencies in essential minerals.

We even wrong in believing that the soft drinks help us to digest. Cook the food too long destroys the nutrients and their enzymes. Raw foods are digested more easily, because they contain enzymes. Eating fruits, vegetables and local foods and of the season respects the alternation in our organic cycle. The treatments Thermal food would distort the proteins that would no longer be recognized by our system.

Once the enzymes are exposed to the temperature, they are no longer capable of fulfilling the function for which they were designed. The food products cooked contribute to chronic diseases because their content in enzymes is damaged. The digestion of cooked food uses of metabolic enzymes to help digest food.[108]

Supplements with enzymes help digestion and the absorption while preventing the degenerative diseases. There is therefore a link between the enzyme deficiencies and the autistic symptoms.

For children with autism, enzymes would not replace the regime GCMS (without gluten, without casein; today also SS [without soybeans]), they would however to prevent possible accidental exposures by reducing the associated symptoms.

The pasteurized dairy products no longer contain the enzymes which would help us to digest and assimilate their nutrients including calcium. The lactose intolerance did not exist or very shortly before the pasteurization. "In reality, 70 per cent of the world population does not produce enough lactase and therefore has various degrees of lactose intolerance."[109]

"About 80 per cent of illnesses are born of a disability of the digestive functions."[110] The digestive abnormalities and immunity go hand in hand, since the destruction of the digestive enzymes by heavy metals weakens the immune system, which works a lot with the intestines.

"The absence of cooking preserves vitamins, omega-3 and most of the antioxidant molecules."[111] The modern diet deficient creates to chronic inflammation by a lack of vitamins, minerals and essential fat. It is therefore necessary to eat foods alive and avoid eating in a same meal of food incompatible and respect their natural form.

The flora and fauna intestinal diseases

Do not destroy the balance of the intestinal ecosystem. A poor power supply from the industrial food destroys the flora. The microorganisms acquire more virulence with an intestinal flora disrupted. The viruses of the vaccines would become even more virulent with the use of antibiotics. The immune cells move along the intestinal mucosa.

"We need to ask the question of the vaccination before the age of 6 months, or the average age of the Intestinal maturation and immune systems correct of the baby."[112] the intestinal flora appropriate is assaulted by antibiotics and vaccines, which leaves place to a flora disrupted.

The result will be a series of infections treated often by a series of antibiotics that will damage even more the intestinal flora of the Child and its immunity during the same period. However, a child whose immune system is compromised does not react to vaccines as planned. In most cases, vaccines increase the damage immunity and are sources of chronic viral infections and persistent.[113]

The intestinal flora balanced helps the immune system to become mature. Therefore, a intestinal dysbiose night to the immunity. It should avoid to give antibiotics unnecessarily to children in the bottom age.

The intestinal microorganisms absorb any iron creating of the anemia. The brain has need of this mineral. The dysfunctions in the brain from a metabolic imbalance in which the source can be found in the intestines. "Indeed, the clinical signs of a dysbiose (intestinal flora abnormal) are present in close to 100 per cent of the mothers of children with neurological problems and psychiatric."[114]

It is an established fact that the antibiotics significantly damage the intestinal flora by destroying in the intestines of colonies of beneficial bacteria. At the age of 16 years, or sometimes even earlier, these mothers are seen prescribe the pill that they will have taken during a number of years before birth. The contraceptive pill also has a detrimental effect on the beneficial bacteria of the intestines.[115]

It is the same concerning certain drugs such as antidepressants. The intestinal flora of the child will influence its health throughout his life and he inherited this flora of his mother. Some good microbes emit enzymes which also help us to digest. A intestinal flora balanced plays a role in the digestion and absorption of nutrients. The Flora has also an impact on the lymphatic system.

The difficulties of learning comes from nutritional deficiencies, which are derived from digestive disorders caused by an imbalance of the flora. An intestinal flora in health product of antibacterial substances, antiviral, and antifungal, as well as a substance that protects the wall of the intestine. The flora and the mucosa acting together. If there is a problem among a, it causes a problem in the other.

"By lack of beneficial bacteria, the digestive system, instead of being a source of nutrients, becomes a major vector of intoxication for the body."[116] For example, the bacterium Clostridium exudes a neurotoxin. Its presence, like that of the yeasts, has been favored by the antibiotics which it is become resistant. Feed our children with organic meats would help them to make fewer repeated ear infections. We could consider the antibiotics as a substance that destroys the life.

"The quantity of immune cells present in the intestinal wall is such that the intestine can be considered as the first immune organ of the organization."[117] Then, such that the would have if well described Dr. Wakefield, the vaccine of measles abyss the intestinal wall, therefore it is an attack on the immunity. The immune system tract produces antibodies when the digestive tube between in contact with harmful bacteria, viruses or parasites. The intestinal microflora protects us in stimulating and strengthening our immune defenses. It should therefore not disrupt the intestinal ecosystem. In addition, it seems that a delivery by cesarean section will slow down the installation of the intestinal flora, which will revolutionize the digestion and the immunity of the child. When the absorption is disturbed, it results in a poor assimilation of nutrients and the child is at risk to suffer from nutrient deficit giving him, for example, difficulties in concentration and learning.

The pH: acid or alkaline?

The pH of our body as well as that of our blood would become too acids with the time. A land acid contributes to the development of yeast and intestinal parasites, and promotes the establishment of bacterial and viral diseases.

Dairy products acidifieraient our blood pH. The calcium from our bones is released to Combat the excess acidity. "The research shows that the countries where populations consume the most dairy products have the highest rates of osteoporosis."[118]

The intolerance to gluten or to dairy products as well as their normal consumption create a small intestine acid, while its usual pH is alkaline, which explains the emergence of yeasts, which have become our main host, but not the most innocuous. The Candida albicans would also have a role to play in some cancers.

We just less dependent on sugar whose love the yeasts if we consume less gluten. The yeasts love the industrial food refined. It is better to do not feed if one wants to get rid of it. The sugar is also an acidifier. "Any excess of sugar or lack of fiber acts on the flora of fermentation, the excess meat on the flora of putrefaction."[119]

Red meats make the intestine acid. The lack of enzymes and good bacteria results in an excess of fermentation and putrefaction. Food badly digested can putréfier, create toxins and clog our intestines by covering their walls of a layer of waste reducing still further the absorption of nutrients. These wastes include the intestinal wall of a crust that prevents the absorption of nutrients. All this increases rot gastric acidity. Of Cancer cells grow less in a land alkaline and provided with oxygen. A form of blood coagulation would come from a lack of oxygen and a pH too acid.

Since the harmful bacteria are also developing in a field that is poor in oxygen, 20 minutes of physical activity per day promote the balance of the intestinal health. In order to increase our alkaline pH, it is enough to avoid the acidic foods and to go to those who are more alkaline. You will find a list of these foods on the Internet. In addition, there are now devices that are restructuring the water of our tap by making it less acid and more alkaline.

The chemistry in our plates

Several Allergic reactions have been observed toward a food additive which would be responsible for the hives, asthma, fatigue and headaches, and which would destroy the vitamin B.

The sulphites, which are part of the nine The most common allergens, are part of the food additives used as agents of conservation. They would be responsible for abdominal cramps, diarrhea, vomiting, puffs of heat, redness. They would be employees also as launderers of food. They would be used also to increase the strength of certain drugs. Conservation Officers and artificial dyes can cause of hyperactivity in some children, those who are the most sensitive.

In fact, new hyperactive children also have food allergies. Since the Food allergies can cause behavior problems, it might well be that the primary diagnosis of disorder of the Attention Deficit Hyperactivity is sometimes established to wrong [...]. Many parents and some teachers are convinced that there is a link between the supply and the disorder of the attention deficit hyperactivity. Perhaps they are better placed than the clinicians to the note. [...] Researchers have advanced the hypothesis that the bulk of the hyperactivity involved in the disorders of learning could be attributed to food dyes.[120]

The human body could collect the difference between a dye natural and artificial. The dyes to candy are implicated in the increase of the hyperactivity.

The food products chemicals to avoid are the following: The thickeners, additives, preservatives, genetically modified organisms, the flavors as well as the artificial coloring. Attention to the mention "Natural flavor", because it can be a cereal that contains wheat and gluten is a source of hyperactivity also.

Is it that the triggering of food allergies is connected directly to the food consumed or to one of its components? For example, an allergy to dried grapes could simply be a sensitivity to sulphites. In their conservation, their transformation and preparation, the foods are more and more distorted. Is it that our system can recognize? Is it that the components can be detrimental to their recognition as well as to their digestion and their assimilation?

The monosodium glutamate (MSG)

The director of an association of autism has mentioned this about the monosodium glutamate: "It is the largest hog producers authorized in the feed." His identity would often be camouflaged under the term of "hydrolysed vegetable protein".

The MSG enhances the flavor of foods by masking an unpleasant taste to make it acceptable. It is a flavor enhancer. It would be added to the power supply for its effects also on the dependency. The restaurants are in would be used in order to maintain their clientele. Even the manufacturers would have allowed themselves to use in their products for the people to choose to the detriment of the other. Have you wondered why you had so often the taste of eat that kind of crispy chicken as often? The FDA would not have issued no limit on the amount that can use the food industry and in the popular drinks, even regarding its use in baby products. It is not surprising to see motorists make the line waiting for the obtaining of a coffee that would be better than elsewhere.

"The monosodium glutamate, when it is administered to women Rhesus (blood H-O Negative), could cause brain damage to their offspring."[121] There is therefore a danger to pregnant women. The MSG would cause several other health problems: injected rats, it has made obese and diabetic. There would also be a link between its use and migraines, autism, ADHD, Alzheimer's, dementia and Parkinson's disease.

"Not only the MSG cause of serious damage to neurons in the retina of the eye, but [...] It has also caused the massive destruction of neurons in the hypothalamus and other brain regions adjacent to the ventricular system."[122] The hypothalamus plays an important role in the organization, because it regulates the growth, the onset of puberty, appetite, sleep, the biological clock and the awareness of itself. Injected to laboratory animals, it has destroyed their neurons. It would cause brain damage, would affect the nervous system and create learning difficulties, behavioral and emotional. Taken at the same time that the aspartame, it would be even more disturbing.

Brain tumors have increased since that this artificial sweetener has been used in the power supply. The monosodium glutamate would be an exciting toxic. It suractiverait brain cells up to their depletion: a kind of excitation sought among consumers. It would produce by following the degeneration of nerve cells, causing their death. It would also affect the spinal cord. It would stimulate therefore extremely cells up to their death. It would then be responsible for the damage to the brain. It would also boost the nervous system that would disrupt the functioning of the endocrine system. It would be responsible for certain sleep disorders. It would affect the production of hormones, which could explain the rise of infertility and the homosexuality, as well as the increase of autism, especially among boys.

The protective barrier of the brain of young children is more sensitive to damage, because it is still at the stage of development.

The MSG would activate the production of free radicals. Adverse reactions after a meal in a restaurant would indicate a sensitivity or intolerance to this product which has long been labeled as "The Chinese restaurant syndrome". Approximately 25 per cent of the population would be allergic to this product.

Among the signs of sensitivity to MSG, found the following ills: rash, intestine irritable, migraine, cardiac arrhythmia, depression, headache, feeling of warmth, lack of attention, fibromyalgia, burning sensation to the lips, in the mouth and in the throat, irritation of the esophagus, heartburn, muscle weakness, tiredness, numbness in the neck, shoulders, arms, chest pain, somnolence, tingling and damage to eyes, paralysis, respiratory disorders, swelling, nausea, reproductive problems, as well as an anaphylactic shock. It would also be in medicines, vaccines, cosmetics as well as in pesticides and fungicides with which irrigating wisely our fruits and vegetables. It is better to turn to a natural food devoid of chemicals, biological therefore and without adjuvants that are rather of opponents to the health.

Of ruminants carnivores

Do you remember the syndrome of the mad cow and scrapie in sheep. It is because that was given of the meat in the form of flour to herbivores. This flour of meat was often end of slaughterhouse waste. Therefore, it could be affected and contaminated. Disrupt a digestive system can therefore cause unrest in behavior related to a certain form of intoxication. Poorly feeding therefore gives health problems.

"Most of the cows receive an inappropriate power [...] including of the genetically modified maize, soybeans GMOS, of animal products (flour of fish), chicken manure, of cotton seed, pesticides and antibiotics."[123] Still today, of the flour of fish would be given to the cows and it would come of waste from fish with a high risk of component of mercury that can be found in the milk. Of herbivores would therefore be fed with fish that may have been contaminated with heavy metals and PCBS.

The animal proteins named "pray" are not destroyed by the digestion of herbivores. The use of fertilizer on the basis of animal meal contaminates water and the soil because it is spread of prions in the nature. The disease can be transmitted to man by the milk since the high temperature would not happen to destroy the prions that have a strong resistance. There is therefore a risk to be exposed well before the onset of the signs in the animal. Prions can be carriers of a particularity protein viral.

"However, it is associated with a degenerative disease of the brain that affects the rights and which is called Creutzfeldt-Jakob Disease."[124] This disease creates lesions of the brain. The brain looks like a sponge, full of holes. Creutzfeldt-Jakob disease would be a human form of the syndrome of the mad cow and scrapie in sheep whose symptoms are strangely similar to a variant of the autism. In animals, the disease is manifested by disorders of coordination with the difficulty to walk and stand, by a disorder of behavior related to a breach of the central nervous system, by a disorder of locomotion and sensitivity. In humans, it is manifest in the dementia, equilibrium disorders, sensitivities, of neuropsychiatric disorders, anxiety, depression, loss of memory.

This disease can also be transmitted to animals by a mite of forage. Is it can be transmitted to man by vaccines grown on infected animals ? That is the question!

The genetic modification

By definition, a GMO is, and I quote, "a body with the exception of human beings, whose genetic material has been altered in a way that does not occur naturally by multiplication and/or natural recombination". It is to levy a gene of a living organism from a plant, a bacterium or a animal, therefore, another species, and of the insert in the genome of another organization. Do we have the right to interfere with the mechanisms of the nature without suffering serious consequences? A gene incorporated in a edible plant can make toxic and the implications for health may appear in the long term.

A gene inserted into a plant GMOS destined for human or animal food risk to produce a toxic substance. In addition, allergies can be triggered by the presence of a foreign gene. "Food allergies are caused by proteins, which are the product of expression of genes. Introduce new genes in a body, therefore new proteins, will increase the risk of allergies."[125]

"We can also, at the time of the insertion of a gene, see the expression of a gene inactive in the body natural which may, in the long term, make a Character allergen again."[126] These changes also cause changes in the sequences of amino acids, which have an impact on the potential allergen. This would therefore reduce the flavor of food as well as their nutrient content. There is a risk that there have serious impacts on human and animal health.

In addition, if the people often consume the same food, there is a risk of it becoming even more allergen because of the period of time that is too short for adaptation. Thanks to international trade, we are exposed to too great a variety of foods that are not part of our culinary customs.

Allergists fear a development of the food allergy for two reasons: 1. It is a substance imported and therefore poorly known; 2. The fact of giving the "milk" of soybean for children allergic to cow's milk protein can make a fear of a awareness among this population.[127]

After the milk, eggs and peanut, soy is ranked fourth in the allergens are most prevalent among children. It will soon be overtaken by the sesame. A gene from the Brazil nut has been added to the soybean to increase its value and protein those amino acids.

To do this, it has added to this soya a gene from the Brazil nut. Laboratory tests have been made to verify that this new soybean was not in the nature of particular allergen, they have all been negative. The Brazil nut is known for its powerful allergenic character, more tests have been carried out, from the blood serum of people presenting this allergy. It was then realized that the people who are allergic to the Brazil nut were also allergic to this soya manipulated. It has therefore never been marketed. This demonstrates, however the low reliability of laboratory testing.[128]

The genetic modification of maize would explain the increase in this new allergy in the population. Our immune system may react violently against the emergence of a plant or be of the animal world manufactured by the man. The genetically modified plants that emit their own insecticide may also cause respiratory allergies that are also on the increase, without forgetting the disturbances of this insecticide food on the intestinal flora.

Therefore, the genetic modification of organisms can trigger allergies. No settlement in the country only requires the labelling of GMO food.

Chapter 10

The Antibiotics

Ear Infections

According to studies conducted in the United States, several children have developed the Autism after having taken much too of antibiotics to combat the repeated ear infections. Behaviors such as hyperactivity, a loss of interest for the immediate environment and a falling asleep difficult would have arisen as a result of these treatments, as well as a regression of the word and a decrease in the visual contact.

"A recent study suggests a link between autism and the Augmentin, antibiotic commonly prescribed for the treatment of ear infection in the child."[129] The mouse who have received antibiotics are isolated from other remain hidden in a corner. The use of this antibiotic would coincide since its introduction in the 1980s with the increase of cases of autism. Some parents have mentioned that they are convinced that the hyperactivity and attention deficit of their child are occurring as a result of catches of antibiotics.

A large percentage of consultations would be for ear infections. Antibiotics are the drugs most prescribed after the antidepressants: millions of orders each year. Normally, ear infections heal on the inside of less than a week, and more commonly after two to three days. The use of a drug against the pain, even as an anti-inflammatory, is more recommended now. In 60% of children, the pain decreases as soon the second day. Approximately 70% of the Ear Infections heal alone without the help of antibiotics. A recent news report aired on a television channel in English Canada showed for the first time also openly in public that there is a link between the intestines and the brain. It has been demonstrated that the massive taken antibiotics for ear infections trigger autism because they destroy the intestinal bacterial flora, while leaving live a harmful bacteria and neurotoxic, Clostridium, which produces a form of acid that affects the brain especially if it is nourished with the food she prefers: starches in Basis of gluten and dairy products. ("Autism Enigma", the nature of thing, David Suzuki, CBC.)

Previously, the antibiotics were prescribed in an automatic way. However, most of the middle ear infections will heal spontaneously. It can therefore wait two to three days before prescribing of antibiotics in the children of more than two years, when the symptoms are not serious. A simple redness of the eardrum does not automatically mean that a otitis is present. This redness should be accompanied of liquid behind the eardrum and other symptoms such as fever.[130]

Ear infections are not all of bacterial origin. In the case of a viral infection, antibiotics are not used to nothing, and even less if it is caused by yeasts or food intolerances or by poor aeration of the back of the throat.

Antibiotics are often prescribed for otitis media, but they must not be if the origin of the latter is non-infectious disease. As is the case in 40 per cent of middle ear infections, it should turn to another therapeutic avenue [...]. If the infection was indeed the cause of otitis media, one would expect that the antibiotics are effective in these cases. However, several children with otitis media do not respond to antibiotics.[131]

How can we decide if our child has need of antibiotics just in him looking at the ears of almost without analyzing a culture in advance? The first dose of antibiotics can increase up to six times the risk of emergence of recurring ear infections as well as the need to have recourse to other antibiotics. We are wrong to believe that their use reduces the recurrence, the duration and intensity of the episodes. Ear infections are of various origins and they do not require all the one and the same treatment.

Some data support that the prevalence of food allergies is higher among children suffering from ear infections. A study has shown that half of children with ear infections recurrent serious were allergic to foods and that in 86% of them, an improvement was felt by removing the food in question.[132]

Among the foods most criminalized, one finds: dairy products, poultry and eggs. The allergy to milk, eggs and chicken can come of vaccines grown on these products. During a esophageal reflux (RTN bad), which is a means for the body to reject a food difficult to digest, gastric fluid can reach the middle ear. These food allergies create inflammation to the glands as well as to the Eustachian tube in thus preventing the liquids to drain and produce a congestion of the nose, from where the accumulation of liquid behind the eardrum which subsequently becomes a favorable environment and favorable to the development of bacterial pathogens. The glands adrénalides, accomplices of the immune system, are so swollen that they must sometimes, in the case of repeated ear infections, to be removed in order to allow a better aeration of the back of the throat.

The biomechanical obstruction can be caused also by a bad positioning of the eustachian tubes to the horizontal thus prevents the liquid to flow in the throat. The abnormal functions of the mechanism of the skull, jaw and neck can be due to injury during a trauma of birth or as a result of a fall. These bad positioning also result of inflammation. The nerves can thus be irritated by the vertebrae causing inflammation which obstructs the ducts. Of the natural products offered by a naturopath can help to strengthen the immune system, as well as visits to an osteopath or a chiropractor. Remove the allergenic foods such as dairy products, sugar and eggs while giving vitamin C, zinc, probiotics and echinacea can help amply.

If in animals as the rabbit and the dog, ear infections can be caused by the presence of yeast, it is the same for the human since the presence of the thrush on the language demonstrates that the intestinal yeasts can reassemble the esophagus, the throat, the nose. In addition, certain harmful bacteria are friends of yeast and one draws the other. The exaggerated use of antibiotics is responsible of the thrush (language white), therefore of ear infections also.

The autistic children suffer from two to three times more often of ear infections that the children not with Autism During the first three years of their life. Approximately 5 per cent of the children who take antibiotics will suffer from food allergies, but also respiratory. These allergies are frequent during bowel disorders. Of antibiotics given to children of less than one year would accentuate the risk to suffer from asthma, especially if they are under the age of six months. The risk is higher among the children of less than three months.

"These drugs would destroy microbes important in the resistance to asthma and other respiratory diseases among young children."[133] The asthma would be connected to the intestinal flora. Approximately 15 per cent of the children who take an antibiotic will have diarrhea. Antibiotics are the cause of stomach problems. They would be the same of the triggers of the celiac disease. The antibiotics and the antidepressants may inhibit the action of certain enzymes leading to food allergies and triggering the intolerance to gluten and dairy products.

Vaccines of new pointing of the Finger

Knowing that the animals as the cat, dog and the rabbit can suffer from ear infections, and knowing that the virus for the manufacture of certain vaccines are grown on these animals, I wonder if it is possible that the animals have transmitted as well ear infections to the man. If this is not the case, some live virus vaccines are the triggers of ear infections in man. If the pertussis may cause otitis media, what is his vaccine? It is the same for varicella. Measles can cause coughing, the irritation to the eyes and the runny nose, which can clog and cause the inflammation to the eustachian tubes leading to ear infections.

"A vaccine, as any medication, is able to cause serious problems, for example of acute allergic reactions [...]. It [the measles] can lead to: an ear infection, pneumonia, seizures, cervical disorders, death."[134]

The mumps, by swelling of the glands, can exert pressure on the eustachian tubes and thus prevent the liquid to flow. Knowing that the MMR vaccine contains live virus, it makes me perplexed and concerned. Some people who are allergic to gelatin (bovine or swine) and to an antibiotic should never receive the MMR vaccine, and 5 per cent of the population is allergic to penicillin. My son who has developed the Autism after the MMR vaccine was allergic to penicillin and to proteins cattle. How many doctors consider this before the injection?

Want to vaccinate a child who is often of ear infections against pneumococcus, whereas it is already under antibiotics, without even knowing if the pneumococcus is the cause, it is assaulting a immune system already weakened. It seems that the vaccines and antibiotics are become a medical obsession, almost a dictatorship absurd and dangerous.

The excretion of mercury

In the pervasive developmental disorders is found the difficulty to evacuate the heavy metals of the body which often remain imprisoned in the tissues. The Antibiotics slow the excretion of heavy metals to a considerable extent. This insufficiency is created by the alteration of the intestinal flora. Mercury may not be excreted from the body by the track fecal, for as much as the intestines and the flora are in good health. Mercury can therefore remain a prisoner in the body as a result of the increased harvest of antibiotics. Studies conducted on rats showed that antibiotics taken by mouth prevented almost entirely the mercury to evacuate the body.

A 2007 study conducted in the Arizona State University establishes that children with autism have higher rates of mercury in the body as the children not achieved. According to the study, children with autism have also been treated more than the other by antibiotics at the bottom age. The use of antibiotics is known to prevent almost totally the excretion of mercury in rats, to cause alterations in the intestinal flora that they cause. Thus, a higher use of oral antibiotics in children with autism has been able to reduce their ability to excrete mercury, which could explain the higher rates of mercury stored in the body of these children. In 2003, researchers from the University of Cambridge, Massachusetts, had already shown that children with autism excrete by the hair of the quantities of mercury significantly reduced compared to normal children. Thus, discard the mercury from its responsibility in autism, as this has been done recently, under the pretext that children with autism do not excrete more of mercury in the hair and the other children, is totally fallacious. Similarly, people with autism have rates of mercury more low in the urine. And for reason, mercury remains fixed in the body, the brain in particular, instead to be excreted. In the light of these studies, we can advance the following hypothesis: children with autism have capabilities of excretion of mercury lower than those of the other children (by genetic predisposition or because of the early administration of antibiotics). The non-mercury excreted is fixed on the target organs including the brain (mercury has an affinity for the nervous tissue), where it exerts its neurotoxic effects.[135]

The inadequacy of the excretion of mercury would be linked to a lack of glutathione accentuated by a increased harvest of oral antibiotics. These are the children who have been treated more than the other by antibiotics which have developed the Autism. A yeast infection also prevents the mercury to get out, because they are used to build a shelter. The pathogenic bacteria also used the mercury to strengthen their protective membrane thus preventing the antibiotics to join them and kill them. The thimerosal in vaccines would thus prevent of antibiotics to be effective and would cause a bacterial resistance triggering of infections to repetition as the ear infections. The Antibiotics therefore slow down the excretion of mercury in a manner to consider seriously. It is stored in the body for up to achieve high levels by accumulation such that in the reminders of the vaccines.

This intensive use of antibiotics has two likely major side effects: 1. The almost total destruction of the healthy intestinal flora, possibly for the benefit of a proliferation of yeasts and pathogenic bacteria; 2. The inhibition of the excretion of mercury, a hypothesis based on a study on rats which has demonstrated that the oral antibiotics multiplied by 10, or even more, the half-life of mercury prior to its extraction.[136]

The antibiotics also have an impact on the liver. A toxicity is done in the digestive tract and all Y organs being linked, including the liver which, by force of congestion, is no longer able to detoxify or to clean the system.

The fever: an ally and not an enemy

The Fever is a sign that some immune mechanisms are activated. The increase in temperature stores the essential nutrients in the liver making them non-available to pathogens who need to develop and multiply. The drugs against fever prevent the immune system to do its work. Fever is therefore a normal reaction and natural body to defend against a bacterial or viral infection. "The presence of fever is therefore a sign of the good functioning of self-defense of the mechanism the body."[137]

Lower fever, is the fight against its own defenses. "The enemies of my enemies are my friends", says a proverb. Hippocrates, the founder of the basic principles of the medicine, said that he had to use the fever: "The fever is witness, but it is not an accomplice." We consider today the fever as an enemy that must be slaughtered at any price while it is our friend.

"We must not turn back the fever by drugs because this could paralyze the natural defenses of the organism."[138] Without the fever, the white blood cells do not multiply not to fight infection. It also eliminates the toxic waste: without it, they accumulate so. A high temperature is necessary to sterilize the germs and prevent to multiply. The Fever is harmless and usually disappears at the end of two to three days. It is very rare that it crosses the 39 degrees.

The human body is equipped with a self-regulating mechanism whose purpose is to maintain the temperature within the normal limits. The hypothalamus [...] puts into action the systems of warming or cooling by sweating, vasodilatation, and chills to restore the body temperature at its fair level.[139]

The fever could be dangerous from 41 degrees if it persists. At the bottom of 39 degrees, the taking of drugs would not be necessary. It is better to lower the temperature of the room, undress the child and put him a wet towel on his forehead; this would suffice to make it more comfortable. Drink a lot of water prevents dehydration. It is more disturbing for babies of less than six months. The Fever is a friend that stimulates the soldiers of our defense system. It must monitor the fever without however hurt him.

"Using too fast of drugs that the font to artificially lower, we replace the aggressors in conditions of development."[140] Give the acetaminophen after a vaccine could prevent the toxins of the vaccines such as heavy metals to be excreted from the body because of the fevers very high are also and often the cause of a poisoning. Unfortunate that we have forgotten to teach future physicians the role of the fever, at least that the trainers are that

98

pharmaceutical representatives. Without the increase in body temperature, the microbes will install and proliferate. Have recourse too quickly to acetaminophen worsens and complicates the disease.

"The Making of Tylenol immediately before or after vaccination has the effect of lowering the immune system and therefore the response to the vaccine, making it less effective."[141] Thus, in this case, bring down a fever after a vaccination may restore the virulence to the live virus for some vaccines. The Fever is a normal reaction, and have after a vaccine is just as normal. If the vaccination becomes less effective, this would mean that these components in Live virus and toxins can become dangerous.

"Give the acetaminophen to a child has a detrimental effect on the immune system of the response to vaccination."[142] A link has been established between the taking of this medication to bring down the fever and pain as a result of a measles-mumps-rubella.

The Autism Journal has associated the use of TYLENOL in tandem with the administration of the MMR vaccine to an increase in the risk of autism. The acetaminophen after vaccination measles-mumps-rubella has been linked to a higher risk of 6.11 times in autistic disorders in children aged five years or less. In contrast, the use of ibuprofen after the MMR vaccine is not associated with autism spectrum disorders.[143]

It is better to have recourse to the ibuprofen (Advil). "The exponential growth of the incidence of autism has begun to happen in 1980 when acetaminophen began to replace aspirin for infants and young children."[144]

The aspirin, associated with Reye's syndrome, is another example of the early marketing of pharmaceutical products dangerous without the assessment of the risks and consequences in the long term.

The use of acetaminophen among pregnant women may be associated with autism from birth. Why guard-t-on this product for sale free? And why the doctors would continue-they of the Advisor to parents after a vaccine if the child cries or fact of the fever? Do they know what they are doing? Are they aware? The rate of autism would have increased in the United States when the acetaminophen would have replaced the aspirin, but the rate of autism would have also declined when this product has been removed from the market between 1984 and 1989 to the cause of the deaths caused by cyanide poisoning. It also accuses the acetaminophen to be responsible for allergies, asthma, the rhinoconjonctivite and eczema.

"Use of acetaminophen can damage the liver and its ability to detoxify harmful compounds."[145] During a disability in the sulfation in the liver, acetaminophen oxidizes and would become toxic. Use of acetaminophen would exhaust also the glutathione which plays a role in the detoxification. "The liver metabolizes acetaminophen in a toxic metabolite [...] which can damage the cells of the liver by depriving them of glutathione."[146]

If the liver is exposed to a toxicity to heavy metals, acetaminophen would then become a poison that can damage the liver. The hepatotoxic damage may be irreversible, cause a transplantation or death, because the acetaminophen intoxication would cause lesions in the liver.

"The use of TYLENOL inhibits the process which have evolved over millions of years to protect against the attacks microbial and interferes with the immunological development normal in the brain resulting in neurodevelopmental disorders such as autism."[147] Therefore, each time that the fever is defused, this lengthens the time of the disease, the time of the suffering that is connected as well as the time of the cleaning. The increase in body temperature helps the lymphocytes to reach the site of the infection and the fight. Certain enzymes in this fight are necessary, but are only produced when the degree of body heat allows. When the fever Monte, it is a sign that our immune system works well. The drugs against fever prevent the immune system to do its work logically. The microbes remain, dirty the field more, which can lead to chronic and degenerative diseases.

It is the same regarding cancer who does not like the high temperatures. The rate of cancer has increased at the same time that our pharmaceutical obsession to want to absolutely lower fever as soon as its appearance. Very high temperatures, beyond 40 degrees, allow the production of active lymphocytes to fight a tumor. The healthy cells are resistant to the rising temperatures. To more than 41 degrees, the cancerous cells die.

The antibiotics affect the immune response, even that acetaminophen which would be linked probably in breast cancer.

"The consumption of antibiotics could be associated with a slight increase in the risk of some cancers."[148] regularly take antibiotics indicates a weak immune systems which leads to inflammation, which can trigger the process cancerous. Some antibiotics are detrimental to the intestinal flora, which plays an important role in immunity.

The dangers of the antibiotic resistance

The misuse of antibiotics makes the bacteria resistant to treatment. The bacteria can produce an enzyme which is opposed to the antibiotic in the Amending chemically. The resistance to the antibiotic occurs when the bacterium is in contact with heavy metals even at relatively low concentrations. It is very contradictory knowing that some antibiotics contain arsenic and that the bacteria feed on it. The contact of the heavy metals, the bacteria can activate a certain gene that tightens its cell membrane preventing the product of the reach and kill them; that is why it is necessary to avoid the use of antibiotics at the same time as the vaccines. The overuse of antibiotics can therefore cause a bacterial mutation. The resistant bacteria multiply, which prevents the complete healing.

The bacteria are fairly cunning to produce germs more powerful, which cancels the positive effect of the drug. The first mission of antibiotics is in decline since it is used as a preventive measure when we should employ them as a last resort when all other resources have nothing given. A dramatic result to the result of the massive use and reckless of antibiotics is to foster the development of a kind of microbes which is less vulnerable to treatments.

The bacteria and mold that were before benign can become dangerous, which was unknown before the arrival of the antibiotics.

When prescribed antibiotics, thought must be given to the dangers that can arise from it, because it is possible that they may affect society and the patient himself. The emergence of new resistant microorganisms and their proliferation constitute a significant danger to the public health. The superinfection is usually due to the deletion of the organizations that normally come in fight against the uncontrolled multiplication of resistant organisms found in the body of [...]. Many fatal cases have been registered.

Of antibacterial cleaning products are unnecessary and harmful outside the hospital. The Antibiotics do not create fair to new breeds of microbes, they generate secondary effects. The Ammonia caused by the fermentation of the antibiotic could induce a poisoning to urea (waste of the contents of the body).

The poisoning to the urea is characterized by neurotoxic effects on brain tissue and corrosive on the digestive system. The symptoms include colic abdominal pain, bloating, diarrhea, tremors, an alteration of the coordination, weaknesses, the loss of appetite, as well as other signs often present in the tables of neurological toxicity. In addition, the poisoning to the urea can disrupt the cells responsible for the secretion in the small intestine. Children with autism show them also Symptoms neurological both that the digestive system.[149]

There have been several deaths by blood poisoning in hospitals where it was used a lot of penicillin. People die more often of sepsis that prior to the use of antibiotics. According to the Larousse dictionary, sepsis is defined as: "General infection due to the outbreak in the blood of pathogenic bacteria..." In 2007, 3.6 per cent of hospitalizations have been due to adverse reactions for a single drug in France. We must be more careful before to prescribe psychotropic drugs, antibiotics, analgesics and anticoagulants. The increase of the resistance to antibiotics is responsible for therapeutic failures and many deaths.

"An American study has shown that more than 50 per cent of hospitalizations in the United States were due to the secondary effects of drugs (approximately 100 000 people per year, including 3000 deaths)."[150] Often, the errors are caused by too great a mixture of drugs which interact with each other and against each other; for example, antibiotics interact against the effects of the birth control pill. There is also the bad orders for diagnostics distorted, dosing errors of pharmacists and the non-compliance of the indications by the patient.

"There had, according to the French Ministry of Health, 128 000 hospitalizations and 8000 deaths annually by the sole fact of bad drug interactions."[151] We are intoxicated by the pharmaceutical companies to the point of be blinded? The doctors put the blame on the back of the self-medication and the use of natural products while they allow themselves to prescribe more 10 drugs to a same patient knowing very well the risks of negative effects of drug interactions after the fourth prescribed drug.

Antibiotics are used universally and without discernment to come to the end of any kind of infection, even the least important. They have revolutionized the way to treat. The generation of physicians out of the university since their discovery can not imagine that we can practice medicine without these antibiotics. But their widespread use has had serious disadvantages. The bacteria are resistant to better and better and the diseases have become sensitized to allergies to their use. If the antibiotics had only been used in cases of serious infection, instead to be employees in all minor diseases, the serious infection caused by a bacteria already immune would then be less serious; and allergies to antibiotics much more rare [...]. However, while the attention of physicians is drawn on the need not to use antibiotics that wisely, the farmers are encouraged to use more and more, not only for the care of their animals, such as cows severely affected, but also by adding each day in the food for the animals of lesser value, such as pigs and poultry, to accelerate their growth or to preserve them longer of infectious conditions and unhealthy in which they live. This widespread use of antibiotics in agriculture is likely not only to increase the number of varieties of bacteria in food, but even to launch on the market of foods containing antibiotics. Milk is a striking example of food contaminated by antibiotics. Antibiotics kill bacteria while the latter warn, by their odours or by their colors, that the food is corrupted. But they will not kill the fungi or salmonella that poison the food. These two agencies develop sneaked in foods which, having been treated with antibiotics, will always appear to be costs. This would be a sufficient reason to prohibit the addition of antibiotics in food.

It includes more why the milk of cow can be a cause of repeated ear infections. Even if this is not allowed supposedly on Quebec to give antibiotics or hormones to animals for slaughter, certain meats and dairy products come from the provinces of the West or of the United States where these practices would be permitted and are found on the shelves of our supermarkets and then in our plates. The antibiotics added in animal feed are responsible for the emergence of bacteria resistant to antibiotics used for treatments humans. In 1999, the Commission of Agriculture has prohibited the use of four types of antibiotics for humans in the feeding of the animals.

"The food use of antibiotics improves from 3 per cent to 7 per cent the speed of growth of animals."[152] The breeders claim that they use of antibiotics in the aim of preventing certain infections, while it is well known that it is for the animal to grow two to three times faster. Antibiotics have the dual function to be used as a promoter of growth. Why Farmers Do they not eat themselves an animal that they have fattened as well, but rather a high beast of a a natural and organic way?

The action on the microbial flora of the digestive tube of the animal product of the metabolic changes that can be also a hormonal disruptive for the beings that feed on his flesh.

We can say today that the danger of the use of antibiotics in animal feed comes not from the inferred residues by the consumer, but rather of the risk of direct selection in the digestive tract of the animal, of resistant bacteria likely to be transmitted to the man through the food or to transmit their resistance genes to the human intestinal flora.[153]

The Ministry of Agriculture had drafted a scientific report in 1995 which evokes the danger to human health of the use of antibiotics in the food of the poultry and pigs. "The Public Health Agency recommends that Canadian citizens to pressure from farmers and the relevant political authorities for the use of antibiotics in agriculture is limited."[154]

Household products for cleaning and perfumes also affect our immune system. In all cases: "It is the dose makes the poison." The antibiotic is a drug. As with any medication, it would also be a poison whose dose is calculated in order to make Inactive an infectious agent while preserving the life of the patient, but we do not know that all its harmful particles are additive with the use. The arsenic would be used in the poisons to rats. And yet, chickens, in addition to breathe the ammonia and dust faeces of barns, would be fed with chow containing arsenic as an antibiotic to that their flesh keeps longer by avoiding the proliferation of salmonella.

The antimicrobials to basis of arsenic are used in large part from farms in poultry and pigs on the global plan (more than 70% of the U.S. poultry is Nourished each day of antimicrobials to basis of arsenic). A group of antimicrobials used for the promotion of growth contains components of organic arsenic.[155]

Approximately 70% of the antibiotics used in the United States are intended to supply the chicken and beef, and this, even if they are not ill. The very large majority (90%) of the arsenic given to livestock would be converted by the animal in a toxic form. Burn the remainder of the carcasses would release of gases of arsenic. This heavy metal would be also present in the fertilizer. Arsenic is found in their manure that is extended in the fields and which, subsequently, contaminates the courses of water and groundwater. The application of manure and fertilizer would therefore increase the rate of arsenic in the water disrupting the sexual hormones of fish. Chicken manure spread on agricultural land affects the development and reproduction of fish, because 75% of the arsenic content in the manure from poultry and pork eventually ends up in the course of the water. The bacteria present in the water feed of arsenic that became soluble in his contact.

"An addendum to basis of arsenic used in the feeding of chickens can cause health risks for humans who eat the meat of chicken."[156] The Antibiotics contained in the meat of animals that we consume can weaken our own immune system making us more vulnerable to infections.

"Many antibiotics are likely to cause kidney damage."[157] The antibiotics can cause hepatic impairment, a slowdown in the elimination of bile and yellowing of the teeth. They would be hazardous in neonates and premature infants since their enzymatic system and immune systems is immature and in full development. The use of antibiotics could prevent these two systems to develop normally.

"Several experts believe that the rise of allergies in modern societies can be explained in part by the omnipresence of antibiotics in the environment. Some scientists believe that the pervasiveness of antibiotics could contribute to this dysfunction of the immune system."[158] The risk of toxicity, effects on reproduction and on the progeny have been noted.

Chapter 11

A multiple intoxication

There has of the disturbance in the air

The environmental factors began seriously to be regarded as playing an important role in the emergence of the autism and other chronic diseases.

"In effect, today, scientists are becoming more and more concerned about the effects of chemical pollution on the health of the most young people."[159] Of disrupters accuse the pollution in different forms to be at the origin of the increase of certain diseases among young people such as allergies, autism and cancers. The pollution of the atmosphere and of the immediate environment would be at the origin of a certain form of poisoning. Four children who lived in American cities too polluted suffered from autistic disorders. When these families are gone to establish in the campaign, several symptoms have decreased and others are completely missing.

"In the neighborhoods polluted cities such as New York, mothers have more risk to the world of children who will have problems of cognitive development and a delay of learning."[160] Why found-t-on the highest rate of autism in the most industrialized countries? Pollution alter the climatic conditions which, becoming disturbed, font fluctuate oxygen concentration, because the transport of molecules of oxygen is disturbed by the pollutants in the air. The oxygen is the origin of life on earth. Our ancestors breathed, 35% of oxygen. Today, we do not breathe that 18%. The most polluted cities may contain no more than 12%, while 10% of oxygen is necessary to maintain the life on earth. The oxygen has decreased by 50% in the course of the water. The brain needs a good source of oxygen as well as all the cells of our body to function well, and we offer him, at the place, of pollution in all its forms.

The brain cells are greedy in oxygen. Our brain uses 20% of the available oxygen in our body to respond to its need for energy. The decrease of oxygen on the cerebral plan because a mental fog, concentration difficulties and cognitive disorders. The lack of oxygen because of unrest in the heart rate, which in turn decreases the intake of oxygen to the cells, which have need of oxygen and nutrients transported by the blood; the latter is then responsible for toxin, which slows down the blood circulation. The decline in the blood pace weakens the immune system which may not therefore not fully to fight against these toxins. The omnipresent depression which is on the rise among the population would come from modern to a decrease in the blood circulation and the brain.

Therefore, the availability of oxygen in the air is reduced because of the presence of the pollution. The brain then becomes saturated by all these toxic substances too many in the blood, which blocks its mechanisms of normal operation. The oxygen contributes to the proper functioning of all systems of the body. The toxins present in too large quantities in the blood slow down the operation of certain glands including the thyroid (problem found in the autism) and adrenal glands.

"The oxygen is an agent of detoxification very powerful and when we lack, the toxins accumulate and deprive our body of its vital energy. The oxygen helps the lungs to dispose of large quantities of metabolic waste gas."[161] Our cells can therefore run out of oxygen if there is too toxic gas. "The worst kind of free radicals free toxic in the human body is formed of compounds that come from the exhaust gases of cars."[162]

The decrease in oxygen allows toxins to take their place giving the chance to free radicals to cause damage to the cells. The pressure of oxygen does not decrease only on the plans of the lung and blood, but also on the muscle plans, nervous and cell. Mitochondria are the power plants of the cells and they need oxygen to better accomplish their work. Autism is also a malfunction of the mitochondria.

If a cell lack of oxygen for more than three minutes, she dies; and nerve cells lost would not occur in the future. However, the exercise or therapies in hyperbaric chamber would promote the formation of new nerve cells in which new neurotransmitters, which would improve the concentration and memory. A brain better oxygenated is more alert. This improves the cognitive functions as well as the intellectual performance and physical.

The physical exercise could therefore help children with a Attention Deficit Disorder with or without hyperactivity, since the drug most popular for countering this problem would replace a substance produced by the brain when it is well oxygenated and well fed: dopamine.

A change in the pace of blood as well as its concentration in toxins deprive the brain of essential nutrients. Our habits of modern life and sedentary cause an oxygen deficiency and play a role on the plan nutritious. Approximately 95% of the retained energy in our diet has need oxygen to be released and then used. The pancreatic cells private in oxygen would contribute to the development of diabetes. We are doing less and less of the exercise and oxygen promotes the absorption of nutrients. A large quantity is required to intestinal cells to promote a maximum absorption of all nutrients found in the food. The exercise increases the intestinal absorption of vitamins, minerals and essential fats.

"If the oxygen is not present in sufficient quantity, there may be a loss of absorption ranging up to 70%, resulting in a proportional slowdown of metabolism."[163] In addition, the nitrate consumption would decrease the transport of oxygen in the blood to cells and organs. The deficit in clean air and healthy would contribute to obesity which is also a scourge on the rise since the presence of this important element promotes the elimination of fats. If the essential fats such as omega-3 oils are less absorbed, this affects the delivery of oxygen to the cells. It is then that the bad fats take the place of good fats, which causes a restriction of the cells. The toxins are stored in the fat.

The toxins would be imprisoned in our fats; this would be a way that our body uses to protect our vital organs of toxic elements. The oxygen contributes to the elimination of waste, facilitates the use of sugars and fats, transforms our energy supply, which increases the immune functions and our tolerance to infections. The oxygen helps the immunity to function better.

Yeast infections such as that of Candida albicans to develop more easily on a Body field poor in oxygen. Their presence can damage the cells and decreases the intestinal absorption as well as the functions of white blood cells (antibodies) and red blood cells (nutrients and oxygen). The lack of oxygen acidifies the body. The intestinal yeasts and cancer cells love the land acids for S install and develop. The acidity of the body also destroyed the muscle tissue that can lead to disorders of coordination.

The presence of a high enough rate of oxygen also helps to combat cancer cells. These are anaerobic, whereas normal cells are aerobic. The fermentation of sugar (acidity) has replaced the presence of oxygen in the cells.

"Cancer could not develop in an environment rich in oxygen."[164] This is ignored in the medical system that puts the before the treatments in the chemotherapy which would further weaken the immune system thus creating new recurrences. The lack of oxygen would be at the origin of new diseases in scourge: chronic fatigue, insomnia, migraine, circulatory problems; behavioral disorders, digestive and respiratory. It weakens the physical and intellectual performances. It creates an increase of free radicals, toxins, stress, the harmful effects of drugs, and it increases the recovery time after a intense effort as well as the period of convalescence after an injury or illness . It decreases the brain functions related to the concentration and the functions of the liver in link with the detoxification.

Various forms of pollution

Several kinds of pollution exist: the one that is in us (internal) and that which is around us (external); voluntary (human activities) and involuntary (natural disasters such as volcanoes and forest fires). The quality of the air, water, soil and food is deteriorating. There is also the chemical pollution drug,, industrial, agricultural and agri-food, as well as the visual pollution and sound. This is all part of the environmental pollution and constitutes the elements of stress on all agencies.

A bad power supply, pollution of the air, the water as well as the stress are factors favoring the accumulation of large quantities of the toxins, waste acids which are found in the fat cells, joints, muscles and in some organs such as the liver and the kidneys. These toxins impede the proper functioning of the body, which creates an environment conducive to the development of disease, allergies and immune system problems. The waste acids are attacking the joints, tissues, to muscles and glands.[165]

The stress of daily life as well as the pollution of the environment in general are heavily deplete the resources of our body in its capacity of adaptation. We are wrong to believe that humans will be able to adapt to the pollution, except those who have a genetic baggage sufficiently strong and powerful to not be part of this natural selection, which looks more like a form of genocide. Just in France, there may be up to 3000 deaths per year related to air pollution. In the world, 3 million people died each year of the suites of air pollution. Why, when the gusting wind, this are not all trees that break or to uproot themselves and fall, but only those who have a weakness often invisible? People believe strongly that our life expectancy, quality of life has increased since decades, that we live longer and in better health, except that...

"Instead of quickly die of an infection such as at the beginning of the last century, we die more slowly, most painfully, more sneaky of degenerative diseases."[166] In addition, the life expectancy has declined significantly since the last years because of the high rate of obesity and cancer.

Environmental pollution has not the effects only on the health of humans, but it also affects all terrestrial and aquatic organisms. Approximately 80 per cent of chronic diseases would be caused by environmental pollution. The majority of pathological conditions would have to cause the environment which the food sector covers 60% of the cases. These pathological disorders produce damage often irreversible caused by the accumulation of pollution in our cells. The degenerative diseases have rapidly evolved since the agri-food industry. Our body has become too acid, while its pH must be more alkaline. It is a collective autointoxication.

"According to the World Health Organization, 80 per cent of chronic diseases (such as arthritis, diabetes, asthma, cancer) can be caused directly or indirectly by the environmental pollution."[167] There is a new way of treating chronic diseases by environmental medicine that helps people suffering from chemical hypersensitivity, which are also part of the occupational diseases related to the work. It would be difficult to otherwise explain the increase in chronic diseases of cause mysterious and unknown, although the conventional medicine categorizes everything it can not explain under the term of a syndrome of any kind such as the "psychosomatic syndrome", which becomes a dump of all that she does not understand.

The autism is triggered by attacks from the environment, which can be considered as a Environmental Illness debilitating.

The first years of the child are periods of very great vulnerability to these chemical pollutants. First, because the system endocrine and immune systems is in place; then, because the child undergoes a neurotoxic load equivalent to adults for a weight and a size well below.[168]

Three hundred chemical substances would have been found in the blood of the umbilical cords of children. The blood-brain barrier is reduced by these pollutants and free radicals. The blood of each individual would contain more than 70 chemicals.

The moment when the aggression environmental product is of extreme importance. Multiple aggressions can give rise to multiple disabilities. If there was no assault important toxic in a child until it reaches the age of three years, his brain and his gastrointestinal tract will be reached a stage of maturation sufficient to prevent that autism to manifest.[169]

The pollution alters the operation of several ecosystems, even than the inside of us. It transforms the climate of the earth while amending also our blood pressure; it would force the immigration of certain animal species as well as the proliferation of pathogenic parasites to the detriment of good bacteria useful to our intestinal flora; and it leads to the appearance of chronic and degenerative diseases unknown and hardly explicable. Pollution is an element which disrupts the balance already preset. It can therefore make lasting changes and unfortunately often irreversible, especially when it is attacking the DNA of living cells. It is said that an environment is polluted when its ecosystem is not to degrade the substances introduced and accumulated in its environment. The organization must be able to eliminate the waste to survive. But it is when these toxic wastes are found in the food and water we consume and which are the elements which, with the air, have allowed us to maintain our species in living up to this day?

All toxic materials in the interior of we blend up to produce an explosive cocktail ticking until a drop make the vase overflow. Some qualify this mixture of real recipe of witch. Here, it is references to the sorcerer's apprentices who have fun without thinking about the consequences. With all the accumulation that is done to the inside of us, the system of some people is no longer able to combat effectively all toxic materials which penetrate in their organization, the least and especially not at the same speed at which they arrive.

The current logic in terms of authorisation for placing on the market of industrial products is the following: a product can be used as long as the population is not seriously affected, even if evidence of its toxicity have been established in the laboratory on the animal. A pesticide will only be prohibited for sale that from the moment where an epidemiological study will have proven its toxic effect on the population.[170]

Have they considered the long-term consequences and disastrous on the generations to come? It has multiplied the chemical substances since the Second World War. They affect different systems (neurological, endocrine, immune and reproductive systems) of same that the thyroid gland. In addition, the degree of security to chemicals is established as if all the world reacted in the same way whereas a person on eight would suffer of hypersensitivity. Individuals are become less resistant. On 18 million molecules, the toxic effect of only a few thousand would be known.

First, let us talk about the air that we breathe. The nitrogen dioxide, these particles from the combustion of fossil fuels, is also an oxidant which, when it is inspired, increases our threshold of sensitivity to viral and bacterial infections as well as our allergic reactions. In addition, when the polluted air is mixed with the heat during the heatwaves, it causes respiratory difficulties. The lungs do not filter the which dioxide ultimately ends up directly in the blood. Those who live near the major road axs develop chronic pathologies. The women who live within 300 meters of a highway or to less than 500 meters from a farm multiply by two their risk of having a child with autism or suffering other disorders associated.

The various forms of pollution entering our system by the pores of the skin, mucous membranes , respiratory and digestive tracts. The injections and drugs are also a source of chemical pollution internal. Irradiation is also a form of pollution because it can produce free radicals.

The electromagnetic pollution of our important environment can interfere with the electrical currents of low intensity of our Organization, and cause adverse biological effects with significant impact on the health: headache, malaise, nervousness, irritability, depression, concentration difficulties, insomnia, decreased immune defenses, acidification of the body, reduction in the secretion of melatonin and, finally, in the longer term, risks of cancer, leukemia, tumors of the nervous system.[171]

For the immune system, it is important to sleep away from electronic devices. The pollution of electromagnetic waves produced by the use of electronic games, the abuse of mobile phones messages and texts, television and the computer cause disturbances on the psychoémotionnel plans and nervous, amplifying the agitation of the neurons, which can disconnect the

111

people of the reality and alter their perception and interpretation of the real world. According to researchers, autism would have increased at the same time that the portable devices. The radiation would prevent our immune system to get rid of toxins.

Heavy metals are become a cofactor of body awareness and the nervous system to electromagnetic radiation. We observe an elevation serious epidemic of autism in children, and the widespread use of electronic and wireless devices could well constitute a factor that has been ignored.[172]

The waves are not just disrupt the orientation of bees. If the climate plays on our mood, imagine the rest. The noise pollution can affect also the health, because it contributes to a form of stress which the latter may in turn reduce the immune capacity as our threshold of tolerance. The noise assaults. The irritability becomes a source of family conflicts and social. Even the ultrasound produce of stress and prevent the reproduction of certain animal species that need to communicate to reconcile, what will other breaches in the food chain. The noise pollution is sometimes so strong that it can make us sick, depression, aggressive, or it causes a loss of appetite and sleep disorders. One sees high orders of sleeping pills and antidepressants in people living near railway tracks and airports.

Our homes include other kinds of pollution. Although dust can contain a tiny part of heavy metals, it remains no less than cleaners contain even more. Therefore, a home too own is much more toxic than a house whose inhabitants are not of the household their favorite pastime. Chemical products to the inside of the household cleaners industrial and can unbalance the immune system, create lesions of the internal organs, while another source of intoxication especially when the components are attacking the liver, which has the function to eliminate them.

Here is a true story. My husband was made with our son to visit friends. Our son had travelled alone to the toilet where he played with a tin in aerosol of a cleaner, disinfectant or deodorant A brand is very popular. It is sprayed the head and arms. The next day, autistic symptoms, long since disappeared, have resurfaced. When I contacted the company, I was told that this product had been tested by the same firm who has authorized the use and marketing of pesticides the most used in the United States. Knowing that pesticides are also pointing of the finger in the emergence of autism: no wonder! In addition, it mentioned to me that the product had been toxic because it had not been used properly. And yet, it is when people breathe its particles in the air or when there is that fall on us and are absorbed by the skin?

If some products have been tested separately, never the interaction between the different substances has been studied nor the long-term impact on generations to come. Of the products become more toxic if they come into contact with other. Several chemical products can be responsible for a disturbance on the plan of the behavior. In a hospital for children, I have even seen the staff to use this product for disinfecting of games. Nobody considers the Chemical hyperactivity in some individuals. We do not use at home that natural products and biodegradable, both for clothing and the household and for the care of the body, and even more for the dishes since the products currents for the dishwasher would be the more toxic.

Indoor air is also polluted by the fumes of the materials used in the manufacture of furniture and accessories, binders, cupboards, washbasins, ceilings, curtains, carpets, elements of decoration, tissues, sofas, perfumes, cabinets which emit toxic gases. The phenol of perfumes would attack the immune functions. The formaldehyde content would be in this toxic gas without color which invades our homes that can cause respiratory disorders including asthma, as well as neurological disorders, such confusion. We are therefore constantly submerged by this gas which is harmful for the Health! The International Center for Research on Cancer (IARC) has classified in 2004 as carcinogenic. It also has neurological effects with the occurrence of headache, nausea, dizziness and a feeling of fatigue. Studies have also stressed its role in the development of allergies and asthma in childhood.[173]

Cell mutation can be stimulated by a foreign substance such as formaldehyde. It can produce anomalies in the chromosomes in some species of microorganisms and insects. But what is in it for us? It could also express a form of genotoxicity on mammalian cells. It creates bleeding from the nose, the irritation to the eyes and the skin, respiratory difficulties. It may also produce damage gastrointestinal, including inflammation, which are at the base of the autistic disorders. It has been recognized as that can disrupt the development of the skeleton and of the brain of some animals.

I have found, during my consultations at home, the high number of children with autism to the interior of the new houses. Would there be a link between formaldehyde found still in the houses and the one who composes of vaccines? Here is the answer that I have found: formaldehyde in contact with thimerosal increases its toxicity.

In the new homes or other places waterproof, significant quantities of formaldehyde can be released by the new carpeting or panels made of wood composite of as of plywood panels, particles or chips, which are used in residential construction, in woodworking and in the manufacture of articles of furniture and decoration. The materials explain in large part the presence in high amount of formaldehyde in homes of today.[174]

The formaldehyde would also be present in some products for personal hygiene including those intended for babies. The Exhibitions The highest meet in agriculture, in the manufacture of resins, plastic and in the agri-food industry. It is found in toys to children as the wooden puzzle facts in plywood, teddy bears, clothing, furniture, hair treatments smoothing, household products, glue, the panels of fibers, paints, adhesives, varnishes, cardboard, paper and in the flame retardants. This substance is carcinogenic and dangerous for the thyroid gland. It would still be used in the construction materials.

"Several epidemiological studies in workers have demonstrated an increased risk of cancer of the nasopharynx, nose and sinuses in workers exposed to high concentrations of formaldehyde."[175] Why is it that a substance also a carcinogen is part of vaccines? For that the companies of chemotherapies do fortune? Cancer, as well as autoimmune diseases including autism and diabetes, can therefore be triggered by environmental impacts such as pollution in all its forms.

Formaldehyde has been declared toxic under the Canadian Law on the protection of the Environment (1999) because it enters the Canadian environment in a quantity or concentration of Nature to endanger the environment essential for the life and constitutes a danger in Canada to human life and health.[176]

The dangerousness and the toxicity of the product increase if the houses are too well isolated, if there is no changes of air, and when the moisture accentuates its evaporation. The heat increases its fumes in the ambient air. Although Health Canada claims that the quantity to the inside of our homes is minimal, but it remains no less than the rate of cancer, especially among children, has increased. It would also be in the coatings of floors in vinyl, most plastics, of household cleaners, cosmetic products, hygiene products, hardening of fingernails and as agents of conservation.

Formaldehyde is used as an agent for the conservation of the corpses; it is ultimately reflected in the nature and also in disinfectants such as those used in the field of health. In hospitals, be used to coagulate as well as in the draining of the waste of samples for analysis that may be found in the environment even if some are incinerated, therefore in the form of smoke also; as cleaning instruments in the sinks with this stream which continues its travel until in nature; as well as in fumigation of mattresses in the purpose of the disinfect.

The people most affected are the employees of the construction, the people working in the medical system, aesthetics, in autopsies and housekeeping.

The toxic effects of these compounds are not yet all known. It is suspected of being responsible for the hypothyroidism and of development disorders of the nervous system (autism, hyperactivity, attention deficit disorder, behavior, etc.). As to the products of degradation that flow from it, such as dioxins and furans, they are regarded as extremely toxic.[177]

The long-term toxicity of flame retardants containing formaldehyde has not yet been documented. These flame retardants are the new contaminants of the environment and yet their use is permitted. They would be used on the clothes of the children, bedding, mattresses, furniture, computers, monitors, television, fabrics and upholstery of the seats of different means of transport, wires, cables, foam, construction equipment, toys, packaging, insulation for the places of difficult access. It is when children chew the fabrics and plush toys? Some of these products also contain bromine and chlorine.

The flame retardants would cause disastrous effects on hormones, the thyroid gland, growth and development. In rats exposed to the flame retardants during gestation have had a disturbed development of their skeleton and their central nervous system. It is also a neurotoxin. The studies that claim the contrary would have been financed by the industry itself of the product.

When stores are trying to reduce the presence of flame retardants in their goods, they often receive the pressures on the part of lobbyists chemicals that exert on them a pressure in accusing them of being influenced by the activists of the protection of the environment. Of neurobehavioral disorders would be connected to the flame retardants. His presence would have been found in the umbilical cord. This would be one of the reasons why all these cords are sent to the laboratory for the purposes of analysis after each birth, and we have never heard of the results. A Swedish study has found of the flame retardant in the breast milk; This product can decrease fertility among women or that of its offspring. The clothes in the friperies would have had the time to evaporate the toxic substances in their fibers.

The plastic which envelope if well our health, our life and, especially, our despair

The black gold, this mineral in the precious time and dirty, door if its name well. The oil is the darkness of the soul of the earth. It is as if we had awakened the demons buried in its depths the most obscure. There were reasons why certain materials were buried in the ground, it was their place and they would have had to stay there, but to the place, we broke the crust of the Earth, this placental membrane protective, to extract its bowels all the shit.

From the scientific point of view, the oil is made up of decomposing organic materials which have not been able to be recycled normally. It comes from the decomposition of the body which have not been able to be digested by the earth. But as for any today, the men consider before all the earth as a resource, as a raw material, in which they serve, exploiting and plundering, in total recklessness. As if everything was their due, without respect or gratitude. The men have turned their backs on the wisdom and the laws of the life. They do not know that the earth is alive, and to tell the truth, this is only of interest not even [...]. In their unconsciousness and their ignorance, scientists play on the sorcerer's apprentices by plunging into the depths of the earth to extract of substances that the latter had yet hidden. The earth is like a loving mother who, without cease, takes the bottom material of man, its waste, its diseases, for recycling. But some of these wastes are so toxic that the earth itself cannot transform them. Then, it stores them and traps them in protected areas and inaccessible. As well, it protects the man of his unconsciousness and allows him to continue to live in the hope that it finds the path of wisdom and the conscience. The oil buried in the Earth is one of the places of storage of highly toxic wastes from the sick psyche of humanity. It is in him that are imprisoned anger, hatred, cruelty, what is really dark and toxic. Thus, through the oil, it is their own anger that they extract and bring home the big day.[178]

We have opened the belly and searched in his bowels to extract the feces. There will be nothing to do so as long as we will be more lovers of the money that the nature. Everything that we makes him undergo returns to us. This are our descendants who, unfortunately, écoperont most of our mistakes. "But this is not serious, say several and especially those who do not have children, we will no longer be there." To the extent that they have a happy life on the financial plan.

"We stifle research laboratories where independent researchers proclaim their disagreement. The PETROLEUM lobbyists and plastics finance themselves of studies for sowing the seeds of discord in the minds to big reinforcement of advertising."[179] of petroleum derivatives would be used in cosmetics, shampoos, toothpastes. They pollute the air, water, soil and our immediate environment.

The plastic poses an ultimate problem when one wants to destroy it. Submitted to the flame, it releases in effect of chlorinated substances which cause the appearance of toxic dioxins for reasons of economic profitability, it does not take the time to test long enough the New Substances placed on the market. However, it often takes many years to realize that a product is toxic. All products whose toxicity is undeniable are prohibited, but they continue to poison us for a very long time, most often through the food chain.[180]

The plastic material has invaded our world by destroying the nature and health by polluting the soil, air and water. Three-quarters of our body are made of water. The water is polluted by various sources of contamination ranging from contagious agencies to sediment and organic matter in passing by the hazardous waste such as heavy metals, pesticides, herbicides, petroleum products and substances emitted by the decaying corpses in the land that contain chemicals, drugs, hormones and antibiotics which may eventually find themselves in the course of water and groundwater. "Chemical substances, in particular present in the plastics, would be in the first rank of the accused for the fall in the quality of sperm (reduced by 50% since 1950) and diseases related to the genital apparatus through the endocrine disrupters."[181] Of Toxic food additives such as lead and cadmium as well as formaldehyde have been added in the manufacture of plastics such as PVC, which would have an impact on the liver, kidneys and bones.

Phthalates are chemical products, which, added to the PVC, are used to make it flexible. Phthalates are not related to plastic and can release and be swallowed by children who suck and chew their toys. The phthalates can cause damage to the liver, the kidneys, the hormonal system that adjusts the growth and the normal development of children. It is found, among other things, in of teethers (to make the teeth), the rattles, but also in all soft PVC toys for children![182]

The intestines, liver and kidneys play a role in the process of detoxification. The liver is the body which must constantly face the many toxins from the outside or produced by the body itself. The liver filters the blood, the product of the bile and enzymes to come to the end of undesirable chemical substances. After having converted a toxin, it must eliminate rapidly from the body and this are the kidneys which is discarded in liquid form. Some toxins have been metabolized by the liver, for as much as all these bodies related to cleaning the body work well, which is not the case for children with autism. The obsolete mechanism of one of the bodies interferes in the operation of the other.

Pcbs if infiltreraient until in the groundwater and also ruisselleraient into our courses of water. They would accumulate in animal fat and human. They would be responsible for part of the births of children widened and mortalities in utero or at birth. In causing liver problems, they are damaging to his work of detoxification. The PCBS would alter the behavior, would cause abnormalities in the immune system, would influence the thyroid functions by lack or excess of stimulation.

"Exposure to OH-PCBS as well as to other toxic products present in our environment could disrupt the neural development and lead to abnormalities of brain development as a disorder of learning, the attention deficit hyperactivity and autism."[183]

A diseased brain led to a degeneration, which induces a senility. The Pollutants exert an action on the factors of degeneration such as gases and heavy metals that attack the nerve cells.

"Among the additives most controversial figure bisphenol A, very present in the food plastics and in particular in 90 per cent of the bottles in 2008. The BPA is suspected to be an endocrine disrupter."[184] Bisphenol A would become dangerous and toxic. It is found in most of the plastic objects: bottles, bottles, helmets, sealants, dentifrices. The universe of the dentition plays a role in our intoxication: amalgam, dental sealants and fluorine. All of the products in which their harmfulness would never have been tested otherwise than on us without our consent and as "guinea pigs involuntary".

"Some plastic bottles release of bisphenol A, a chemical toxic, and more particularly when the container is heated."[185] heated in a microwave, bisphenol A may leave the material and seep into the food. It is also found in food containers like dishes, plastic dishes

118

and the layer of protection to the inside of the cans of food and drink, as well as to the interior of the canned infant milk formula. Even the teats can contain. The Rigid plastics in would also such that the plugs of the Bottles.

The rate of homosexuality has increased because of endocrine hormones and we know that they play a role in autism since this are especially boys who are achieved. "It is the hormonal influence of BPA that raises the controversy. Bisphenol A is a little as of estrogens in humans, it can cause hormonal imbalances. It is also suspected to cause cancers of the prostate and breast."[186]

It would be connected also to cancer of the testicles, ovaries, diabetes, hyperactivity, to Obesity and Infertility. It accumulates in the water through the washing and night same to the breeding of fish, breaking another mesh in the food chain. It would disrupt estrogen, would cause cancer in animals, would reduce the fertility and affect also the functions of the immune system. It would be on the subject of puberty girls early, and since the bisphenol emulates the female hormone, it would therefore contribute to the feminization of boys. Its toxicity would therefore on the reproductive capacity of the animals and humans. It would be at the origin of malformations of male genitals such as penis atrophied, and on the testes, sometimes a single not being lowered.

These endocrine disrupters could cause various problems: first in the genital apparatus (malformation, disorder of fertility, sexual differentiation, precocious puberty, etc.), metabolism (obesity, diseases of the intestine...), the immune system and the brain (conduct disorder, memory, autism, etc.). They also encourage the emergence of cancers, mainly of the breast, prostate or testicles. And its effects would be not only felt in the long term, but also on several generations.[187]

It threatens the survival of several animal species including the human being, by its negative impact on fertility. The girls descended from women in contact with the BPA during gestation have risk of not being able to have children in their turn.

BPA was found in the blood of pregnant women until in the placenta and in the umbilical cord, which alters the development of the fetus. It would amend the development and functioning of cells.

"The EWG indicates that bisphenol A may alter the operation of more than 200 genes, or more than 1 per cent of the whole of the human genome. These genes, indicates the study, control the growth and repair of almost all the organs and tissues of the body."[188] Its impact in autism is explained by its impact on the

119

growth of the cells of the cerebellum. It would thus affect the development of the brain. The placenta may not fully protect the embryo of this chemical exposure to bisphenol A as a pass through the placenta significant has been observed and noted in mice in laboratory studies. It alters the development of the fetus in rats.

The presence of bisphenol A was found in almost all the humans who have been tested for this product in the United States. Be exposed to the quantities relatively low has when even an effect on the behavior and the neurons. Bisphenol A may have contaminated the milk for your baby. Approximately 6 per cent of children fed infant milk formula would be exposed to the BPA at greater amounts of those related to the increase of the aggressiveness and hormonal changes in laboratory animals. The level of exposure is 10 times higher than that allowed.

"Babies fed to the Liquid Milk polycarbonate bottles can consume up to 13 micrograms of bisphenol A per kg of body weight per day. Naturally, children in the spectrum of autism are more vulnerable to environmental pollutants."[189]

Several canned foods contain a high rate of chemicals associated with endocrine brain. "A single portion of these foods was sufficiently charged in BPA to expose a woman or a child to a rate of BPA more than 200 times higher than the standards of maximum exposure laid down by the Government for the chemical products."[190]

Children absorb 12 times more than adults. The BPA would prevent human cells to oppose the oxidative stress that their avoid becoming cancerous. Cultures of cells maintained in life by processes in the laboratory are rebelling to the contact of the BPA. It night to the communication of cells between them. It is a danger to the pancreas, liver, the intestines and the thyroid gland.

In December 2009, a French study carried out by researchers of the INRA concludes for the first time that the exposure to bisphenol A (BPA) has consequences on the functioning tract in the rat. The study demonstrates that the digestive tract of the rat is very sensitive to low doses of BPA, affecting the intestinal permeability, the visceral pain and the immune response to inflammation digestive system. The effects of BPA on the intestine are observed with a dose ten times less than the tolerable daily intake yet considered very safe for the man. This study also shows that the exposure Pre and Postnatal of these animals may weaken the function of intestinal barrier in adulthood.[191]

We know the impact of the intestines and the immune system on the autism. This product exceeds the doses that have toxic effects on the animals.

The rats subjected to the action of the BPA would have indeed shown the behavior changes significant ranging from maternal aggression to the loss of capacity drive, explorers, playful. A failure of social interactions, caused by the impact of the BPA at low dose on the neurotransmitter often incriminated in autism, dopamine, should constitute a track for the researchers. The precancerous lesions and metabolic adds, according to the study, to the assets of BPA, intestinal permeability to encourage the retention of water and inflammatory diseases. The fetus, not preserved, would lose its immune defenses.[192]

The BPA would therefore of brain disorders and intestinal disorders. The precocious puberty, obesity and cancer the consequences would be. The baby milk powder would be a better choice than the liquid, although the infant milk formula used in the under-developed countries has caused lethal epidemics of childhood because the mothers would have used of the contaminated water.

I have a good pipe for you

The intestines do not play a crucial role just in the elimination of waste, but also in the detoxification and the protection of the organism. If the toxins accumulate, the intestinal mucosa will swell and infect. When an ecosystem suffers, this are the other ecosystems that are affected. The human body is an ecosystem that depends on the other.

Humans depend on the microbial communities that the colonize to take advantage of benefits surprising. These include: the extraction of energy of the ingested food, education of the immune system and the protection against pathogens [...]. The antibiotics have not really made service to human health. The evolution has selected these microbial populations who maintain and increase the good form of host individuals and the group as a whole.[193]

The antibiotics would be synonymous with "kill life". An old saying says that the death begins by the colon. The stones to the liver and kidneys, diabetes, gout, hypertension, varicose veins, rheumatoid arthritis, obesity and the psoriasis would be related to intestinal disturbances. This is not for nothing that the cancer the most known is that of the colon. The foundations of health are beginning by the digestive tract. We cannot repair the other systems of the body prior to having cleaned the colon.

121

"Our style of modern life in fact pay the price for our digestive organs of elimination. Refined foods, processed by the food industry, without fibers, animal fat, a lack of exercise and a level always growing of stress all contribute to this crisis of intestinal health."[194]

Our intestine acts a bit like the system of toilet, a septic tank and a septic field. It is the pipe of sewer which evacuates the waste of our body. When there is too much, it blocks and waste repressing toward the inside, which gives the symptoms. When you pull the hunting of water from a cup blocked, it will overflow.

The lymphatic vessels filters the impurities from the blood by ingesting bacteria, the old red blood cells as well as the toxic waste various. It is therefore in the lymphatic fluid that is ramasseraient impurities such as residues of drugs and medicines; the heavy metals and pesticides is store in the tissues.

The intestines of carnivores measure three times the length of their trunk; they are very short so that the flesh is absorbed and expelled before putréfier and produce toxins. The humans possess intestines twelve times the length of their trunk and they are intended to keep the food longer so that all the nutrients can be extracted. The liver of a carnivorous is capable of eliminating ten to fifteen times more of uric acid that the liver of a non-carnivorous. The liver of a human fails to eliminate that small quantities of uric acid, a substance produced by the meat, extremely toxic, which can completely disrupt the organization. Unlike the carnivores, the human does not have the urase, an enzyme to break down the uric acid. A lot of human suffering is directly related to the consumption of products derived from animals, such as cardiovascular disease, certain cancers, pollution, the waste of energy and natural resources such as water and cereals, deforestation, the erosion of the land surface, the famine. We could feed properly all the hungry of our planet if we do not give both place in cattle.[195]

The multinationals of the agri-food industry would encourage overproduction to respond to the offer and at the request of a population that is wasting just as much. The quantity of the products then becomes more important than their quality. Farmers and breeders would thus handle by the large companies such as Monsanto. (The World According to Monsanto is to read a book or a DVD to watch.)

There are farmers and farmers who are concerned about the environment and who would be willing to change their ways, for as much as it gives them openly the necessary tools without their impose things that go against their principles. There are others to which financial values pass in front of the human values. For these people, the money will always be more important than the health.

Of Diseases created by the man

The hyperactivity and attention deficit have not one and the same cause, any such as autism, but rather they are due to an interaction between different factors.

"The environmental stress increases the risk in a child to develop a ADHD due to an imbalance in the neurochemical brain. The exposure to certain toxic substances (alcohol, tobacco, lead, pesticides, etc.) during fetal life would explain 10% to 15% of cases (ADHD)."[196]

The solvents, in particular for children, are very toxic to the body if they are inhaled. They can cause a sensation of drunkenness, a disorder of perception, hallucinations and sometimes even a loss of consciousness, neurological difficulties, behavioral disorders, lesions of the kidneys, the liver, the digestive system as well as the respiratory tract. They cause irritation to the eyes and allergic reactions.

We can find the presence of ethers of glucol in paints to the water that would be toxic to the organs of the reproduction. Despite their dangerousness recognized, their use would not be limited or prohibited. There is no safe solvent. The glues would have a psychoactive effect for children. Some of these products may be responsible for certain congenital malformations.

Most of the solvents would be in part responsible for the False layers. It is found in paints, glues, inks, varnishes, maintenance products as well as in cosmetic products such as those related to the field of the hairstyle. Tens of thousands of chemicals would have been put on the market without that their level of toxicity has been tested properly. Even once they are considered toxic, they remain on the market. The products used in the dry cleaning can cause irritation of the skin and mucous membranes, disorders of the central nervous system and damage to organs. The hypersensitivity of mucous membranes would be triggered by chemicals that are found in the air that we breathe, the water we drink, the food we eat and in the objects that we touch.

The MSG (monosodium glutamate) would also be one of the causes of hyperactivity. Heavy metals are also called to the bar of the accused concerning the emergence of ever-increasing the rate of hyperactivity; it is, among other things, cadmium, aluminum and lead. The lead intoxication may come from the mother through the

123

lipstick which is directly absorbed by the skin, respiratory and digestive tract, as well as in other forms of makeup.

"In a group of children whose levels of lead were particularly high, a therapy of chelation designed to reduce these levels has resulted in a significant improvement of the hyperactivity, impulsivity and behavior and learning problems."[197]

The heavy metals form of rust, oxidize, are transformed into free radicals. Antioxidants can neutralize this oxidative stress. Approximately 10 per cent of schoolchildren are hyperactive, and the yeast infection intestinal diseases may also be the cause for some. "Indeed, many children who have cognitive problems or behavior have an intestinal flora often unbalanced as a result of abuse of antibiotics in the treatment of ear infections."[198]

The hyperactivity and attention deficit often come from a malfunction intestinal tract. The candida, which weakens the immune system preventing the extraction suitable heavy metals, is favored by the oxidation of the organization whose main responsibility are the drugs including antibiotics, infections and vaccines; foods rich in animal fat, starch and in dairy products; beverages such as chlorinated water which absorbs an amino acid important, of fruit juices too sweet, soft drinks too acids; the stress related to emotions, to pollution in all its forms; free radicals; the poisoning to household products and from the office equipment, the environment around the farms and factories without forgetting the various drugs, the magnetism of high voltage lines; Portable devices as well as Microwave cooking. The candida in proliferation produces toxins that can penetrate into the blood stream, spread in all the bodies of the same that in the brain and create a form of autointoxication.

Various factors are responsible for this situation (between 70% and 80% of the world population have a chronic infection by candida), and in particular the modern diet degraded, too refined and too sweet, the exaggerated use of antibiotics, the abuse of cures for the central nervous system (tranquilizers, sleeping pills), the contraceptive pill, the remedies against the ulcer (cimetidine), a concentration of more and more important of heavy metals such as cadmium or mercury (dental amalgam, contaminated fish, pollution of the air, water, etc.), the use in the food field agents of conservation and dyes, the use without limits of pesticides, herbicides and antibiotics in agriculture.[199]

The candida secretes 35 toxins which disrupt the functioning of the brain, the immune system and the other systems of the body. It

124

transforms a substance of the sugar into alcohol which reacts on the brain neurotransmitters causing disorders of memory and concentration, mood swings and irritability. It may change the hormones and stimulate autoimmune reactions, arousing the production of auto-antibodies intended to the organs of the reproduction. The candida causes intestinal permeability, and its passage in the blood is accompanied of neurotoxins that can cause depressions and migraine headaches. It is therefore responsible for the intolerance and food allergies as well as the products which have been genetically modified.

Our organization would have the tendency to reject everything that he does not recognize as natural. Is it that the allergic reactions toward the food could be a response of the system toward the food or rather toward what it contains? We would use food coloring in the meat in order to make them seem more red and more fresh. Although this has been denied by a butcher that I have known personally, I realized by purchasing the ham in charcuterie biological completely which, without nitrites, sulphites, preservatives or colorants, deteriorates and changes color more quickly. "Since the meat is a corpse putrefaction, it was use of conservation officers, of artificial coloring and inhibitors of mold. The sulphites, nitrites and nitrates could mask the smell of the meat in decomposition and keep the pink flesh. This are carcinogenic substances and allergens."[200]

The dyes in fruit juice excite the children more than the juice itself, which would confirm that these chemicals have an impact on the hyperactive behavior of children. Other also advocate the withdrawal of artificial sweeteners and aromas of synthesis. These children often suffer from food allergies as well as children with autism. In effect, the ADHD would be a cousin of autism. In both cases, a nutrient deficit is in question, because the yeasts feed on vitamins and minerals. The candida cause of difficulties the digestive tract while fostering a intestinal putrefaction. Similarly, blood tests in these children showed levels of vitamins, minerals and essential fat abnormally low. They often indicate a low rate in iron. Often, these children have also need magnesium, calcium, B-complex (including vitamin B6) and omega-3 oils and 6. The water filtered by the systems is cleared of its essential minerals. The brain is one of the bodies that are the most in need.

A high level of copper and a low level of zinc lead to hyperactivity. A supplement in pycnogénol and GABA will often help to the concentration. The use of other supplements is suggested as well as a specific diet. Although some criticize this approach, it remains no less than of parents and stakeholders in education have noticed the positive changes with the addition of some supplements and the withdrawal of certain eating habits. The nutrient deficit in our food comes from the poverty of the soil and the treatment of food.

In addition to pesticides and other chemicals added to our food chain, it lack in the fruits and vegetables of the essential nutrients called phytonutrients because they are often picked before they are ripe. These phytonutrients reinforce our immune systems and operate as enzymes helping to the digestion and absorption. Add enzymes to a diet will help often people with learning difficulties and attention because the lack of digestion and absorption is often one of their physiological weaknesses.[201]

Among the list of foods to avoid in children with autism, hyperactivity and learning difficulties, behavioral disorders, obsessive compulsive disorders and attention deficit are: the gluten, casein, soybeans, conservation officers, the flavors and the Artificial dyes including especially the red and yellow, aspartame, stimulants such as coffee and chocolate, carbonated beverages, white flour, white sugar, candy, sugary cereal, non-organic feed, the trans fat, GMOS and junk food. Approximately 50 per cent of children with ADHD are sensitive to food additives (colorants, stabilizers, sweeteners, artificial flavors and preservatives). Studies have shown an improvement of the discipline problems and school performance once the artificial ingredients eliminated.

The aspartame would be a toxic sweetener that would diminish the intelligence and the memory. It also would cause a malfunction of the thyroid gland. In autism, it sometimes found of the hypo or hyperthyroidism. The ADHD also constitutes, in many cases, a disruption of the thyroid gland.

Another hypothesis puts into question a possible malfunction of the thyroid gland. The thyroid hormones are involved in the regulation of substances that modulate the nerve impulses in the brain. Various studies suggest that a slight hypothyroidism of the mother during the pregnancy, may affect the intelligence of the unborn child. It was also observed that 45% to 60% of children suffering from general resistance to the thyroid hormone were a problem of SDA/H. It identifies almost 77 chemical substances that can cause damage to the thyroid gland, including PCBS, dioxins, furans, phenols and several other which were commonly observed the presence in the breast milk.[202]

The deficit of attention is often caused by a too large consumption of starch and sugar, foods whose love the yeasts which when they are themselves excited emit neurotoxins. It is necessary to remove in the first place the foods most recognized to cause allergic-type reactions (corn, milk, chocolate, wheat, eggs, orange, soybean) and combat the intestinal parasites in giving of probiotics.

The health of the brain depends upon the availability of nutrients and its accessibility by the influx of blood. A brain improperly nourished contributes to the decrease of the memory and intellectual capacities, depression and fatigue, disorders frequently encountered in the population today. The degeneration of the brain is also caused by the action of free radicals which oxidizes its cells.

The phosphate would be also linked to hyperactivity even if it is necessary to the growth and the proper functioning of the body; in excess, it translates into behavior disorders. It is the lack of serotonin in that fact that it has recourse also too quickly to the Ritalin.

It should systematically try to modify the diet of children before their prescribe a medication. 75% of children with ADHD saw their symptoms will improve when subjected to a regime to eliminate possible food allergies. Similar results have been obtained concerning the refined sugar.[203]

Poison not just in our plates

If a mother is exposed more than five years for the pesticides, its risks of having a hyperactive child would be multiplied by two. If the child is exposed to organophosphate pesticides during the prenatal period, it would be more vulnerable to the development of a deficit of the attention. The people who are close to the agricultural community suffer more from muscle weakness, mood disorders, depression, difficulties of concentration. Of neurobehavioral disorders and alterations in the performance of the cognitive faculties are many among agricultural workers. Pesticides would disrupt the neurotransmitter responsible for the maintenance of the attention and the short-term memory.

"The brain development in fetuses and young children is much more sensitive than adults to disturbance Chemical."[204] Attention deficit is more often encountered among boys, this assumes that the hormones and their ability to detoxify come into line of account. With the mass arrival of insecticides, fungicides, herbicides, Bactericides and rat poison, new diseases have emerged both in animals and in human beings.

Prolonged exposure [to pesticides] can be related to problems of cancers, disorders of the central nervous system, neurodevelopmental outcomes such as the difficulties of learning, the sensory deficit, delays in development, cerebral palsy, Attention Deficit, Hyperactivity, etc. of researchers would have established a link between the use of these pesticides and the violent behavior of young people.[205]

Pesticides cause chronic health problems. The accumulation in the body creates long-term effects. These products can weaken the different functions while risking to cause damage to our bodies. They would disrupt the nervous systems, immune and endocrine systems. "The carbonates and organophosphates affect the central nervous system. The Possible immunotoxic effects of Organochlorines affect the reproductive systems, nervous, endocrine and immune systems."[206] organophosphates would also create sequelae in immune system. They would not be toxic only for the man, but also for all living beings. And, despite their dangerousness, their use would be permitted and without restriction, the least controlled very closely.

More and more people suffer from chemical hypersensitivity to pesticides. That is why people seek food Biological completely because they suffer from multiple hypersensitivity to chemicals, because they are much more sensitive to low doses of pollutants that are normally better tolerated by the average of the population. Given that their metabolism is slower, 10 per cent of the people suffer from side effects. It is their persistence for a long time in the environment which increases the danger to human health. A bioaccumulation occurs through the years. Some products remain in the environment of 30 to 40 years after their use and often even after their ban.

Among the health problems, we would find, among others, skin lesions, liver disorders, chronic fatigue, a decrease in the memory, the disorders to the thyroid gland, a hormonal imbalance, anemia, respiratory diseases, hepatitis, and sometimes even cancer and deaths as a result of poisoning.

The World Health Organization estimated that 200 000 people are killed in the world each year because of a pesticide poisoning. It thus considers that 3 million people are poisoned each year, a large number of them are children. A study in England and Wales has shown that 50% of the poisonings to pesticides involved children in bottom of 10 years.[207]

The organochlorine pesticides would be most harmful to our health. This would however be among the organophosphorus insecticides that there would have been the most poisonings. The serious poisoning create digestive disorders, respiratory and skin.
This are our children who are paying for our mistakes
The PCBS would impede the functioning of neurotransmitters that are responsible for the connection between the different areas of the brain. Pesticides are also detrimental to the development of the brain of the fetus and children leading to delays in the psychomotor development and to an alteration of the cognitive capacities. The herbicides cause delays of intrauterine growth, a feminization in amphibians, genital abnormalities in children males in more of a deterioration in the quality of sperm and a malfunction of the ovaries leading to infertility; a reduction of the Perimeter cranial, degeneration of the nervous tissues, a reduction in birth weight, a fetal mortality and premature births. They are the cause of false layers, spontaneous abortions; although the latter are more often in women farmers, pregnant women in contact with pesticides have more risk of having an autistic child. The reproductive functions of boys are disturbed in mothers who have worked in greenhouses. They would cause a decrease of testosterone, the length of the penis and the volume of the testes. The damage is irreversible if they take place at the embryonic stage. Young people, their systems are immature, in full development and not yet functional.
"The tests on rats have shown that exposure to pesticides induced a modification of the areas of the brain involved also in multiple sclerosis. In addition, pesticides showed a activity of severe destruction of the gastrointestinal system and causing neurological disturbances."[208]
Among the brain disorders are a loss of sensation to the ends, paralysis and anomalies of intellectual functioning. Three families of pesticides are suspected to create the legacy to the nervous system. Among these would be the organochlorines, carbonates and organophosphates.
Which filter the stimuli to the brain would be defective. A confusion or a fascination installs caused by hypersensitivity or subsensitivity Of the five senses. Of the diseases treated as of psychiatric disorders would indeed that a environmental poisoning. The symptoms related to a poisoning are often considered by the medical system as psychosomatic disorders because the doctors can not otherwise explain that in making believe to their patient

that it does happens that in their head, whose problems of digestion, the pain to the organs and muscles, irritability, asthma, depression, headaches, chronic fatigue...

Even the nitrates that are found in fertilizer can cause a form of leukaemia Fatal in children. The Agent Orange is a defoliant celebrates who has been implicated in physical and mental disabilities and that would have been used by the suite as chemical weapon.

"The consumption of residues of pesticides in food is responsible for 1.4 million deaths from cancer in the space of a generation."[209] Approximately 30 per cent of the pesticides, 90 per cent of fungicides and 60% of the herbicides are carcinogenic. Of the organophosphate pesticides are accused of having caused neuropsychological disorders and neurological disorders to farmers, to their close family as well as to their workers.

"As regards the infections, they would also have the ability to trigger the opposite effect, either to increase the resistance, which increases the risk of autoimmune diseases or allergic reactions."[210] insecticides may therefore be responsible for the increase in asthma and allergies. The immunotoxic would be commonly used in agriculture and horticulture.

More and more evidence attest that the functioning of the immune system may be disrupted by excessive exposure to contaminants in the environment such as pesticides. Disorders of the immune system and alter the capacity of our Organization to defend themselves against the attacks of the outside, particularly against infections, tumors and cancers.[211]

Pesticides can cause disturbances to the lymphatic system and inhibit the operation of the mitochondria, another reported phenomenon in the physical disorders involving the autism. A mitochondrial inhibition may result in the death of cells which even those in the brain, thus creating of lesions, and other bodies because of a lack in energy intake and nutrition.

"Children are more vulnerable to the development of cancers, as a result of exposures to toxic substances such as pesticides, due to the rapid division of their cells, their reduced capacity to get rid of toxins and their great capacity for absorption."[212]

A functioning of the DNA to its point of surveillance because of the flaws in the Cellular replicas. Research have recognized the genotoxicity of the organophosphates which act as a mutagen. They cause mutations in bacteria of our intestinal flora, which would explain a lot of things.

Gastrointestinal disorders can be caused by contaminants of agricultural origin; for example, the liver of poultry of livestock can contain a high rate of heavy metals and carcinogens including cadmium and arsenic. The Vitamin B12, which is normally produced by the intestinal flora when she is in good health, is often missing in most of the children with autism. Of antibiotics, chemicals and surgical interventions to the intestines or the stomach inhibit the absorption of vitamin B12. The cigarette and alcohol are also involved. The slowness of the digestion of meat disrupts the manufacture of this vitamin. The deficit in vitamin B12 can cause of the anorexia, digestive disorders, pallor and severe anemia.

In addition, a refined power supply denatured and increases the need for vitamin B12. Nitrates cause certain forms of cancer as well as comas followed or not by a death.

Nitrite can also react with amines in the stomach to form nitrosamines. These last would have a potential carcinogenic, teratogenic and mutagenic in several animal species, including primates. The cancers most often associated with the consumption of water in which the levels of nitrates are high are those of the esophagus and the stomach. According to other studies, nitrosamines, crossing the placental barrier, could affect the development of the child.[213]

Beings in track of appearance

Some animals are threatened because of all these materials which are toxic for their neurons. If the jellyfish are proliferating in the world, it is because the chemical products may not destroy their nervous system given that they have not. Concerning the disappearance of amphibians and animals that feed on them, the chemicals used in agriculture play a decisive role in their proliferation. Frogs distorted were found in the ditches surrounding the fields of corn and potatoes. Pesticides do not come just to the end of the small creatures. They eliminate also of organizations that are not targeted. Soon, all these products will eventually come to the end of the major bugs also.

There are many types of poisons in the insecticides, but the more dangerous are those to basis of organophosphates which are in fact of nerve gases for insects. But the chemical substances can be very dangerous to humans if insecticides are not used in a proper manner.[214]

Which respects the recommendations related to weather conditions? Especially when I see farmers spread of manure on the eve of a thunderstorm and other who water a field of herbicides when it sale.

The carbofuran kills without distinction earthworms, rabbits, foxes, ravens or eagles. The Raptors die after eating birds, rodents or insects contaminated by chemicals. Even dogs and cats can become ill or die after being rolled in a field freshly treated the carbofuran or after drinking dirty water by the chemical substance.[215]

If the pesticides increase the rate of infertility in humans, they can do so also toward the other living beings. The men exposed to dioxin and furans generate more girls. Since a few years, we also note a feminization of the wildlife: 70% of fish are females. The effect reprotoxique can be observable also among some insects useful for the plantations.

Pesticides can be ingested through the power supply or breathed or absorbed by the pores of the skin. They would affect the eggs of fish and reptiles causing genetic defects that appear later during their growth. The thinness of the shell of the eggs of fish-eating birds would be caused by the ingestion of organochlorine pesticides.

Pesticides do not eliminate just the parasites, but also beneficial insects including earthworms that are so important for the aeration of the soil so that it does not become compacted. This are the earthworms that recycle organic matter thus making available nutrients and soil more fertile to plants. A soil death is a poor soil in microorganisms, in insects and earthworms. "In the 1950s, soils included two tonnes of earthworms per hectare in the fields. Today, there is less than 100 kilograms per cultivated field."[216]

Farewell, my Little Bee

Pesticides are toxic for the development of the nervous system. The neurotoxicity is the mechanism of action of certain brands of insecticides, even those for domestic use, which is the source of neurodegenerative disorders as well as neurobehavioral disorders not just in the target insects. The development of the brain of the fetus and young children can be affected by the many pesticides used by farmers and consumers.

The nervous system of some insects is targeted by pesticides whose organophosphates which interfere in the mechanism. The everything is played in the inhibition of an enzyme which rule the transmission of nerve impulses, which can no longer go to the muscles, can cause paralysis, a slow reflexes and confusion, symptoms observed also in humans.

"To the extent that many of them are toxic to the brain of insects, it is very likely that they are also for the brain of humans."[217] The antimoustique sprayed in residential areas, parks and around schools would be equally toxic. Of the students have been evacuated for intoxication or poisoning to the organophosphates. Bees are just as affected by the insecticides. We have been witnessing since little to a new phenomenon: the syndrome of collapse of colonies of bees. In 2008, 36% of them were missing. Today, this figure had increased to 90% in some regions. Approximately 80% of the plants of the planet depend on pollinators. Albert Einstein had predicted that if the bees disappeared today, this would be a world famine in four years. In the era where the earth is overcrowded, this is not the time that such a thing happens!

The hives could be contaminated by the organochlorines. The bees who succeed to return to their hive without having been too disoriented poison all residents. A molecule of an insecticide which seeds are coated is pointing of the finger by beekeepers as responsible for the decimation of bees. Pesticides may be the cause of the excess mortality of bees. Many of the agencies are in a different environment from that of their ancestors.

"Since thousands of years, the bees are very well accommodated of parasites and diseases; what is new is this which has been introduced by the man: the neurotoxic."[218]

If the bees can not return to their remains, it is because it would have happened something in path. Some insecticides can confuse, same as the electromagnetic waves of our portable devices. The overuse of pesticides develops the resistance of certain pathogens which may therefore promote a fungal infection, where the link with yeast infections of our own intestines. If the bees are resistant poorly to a parasite, a bacterium, a virus or a fungus, it is because their system has been weakened by something else. Their mechanism of defense is decreased by insecticides which act as immunosuppressive drugs. Then, it is very likely that the pesticides also affect our immune system, also invaded by the yeast resistant. The immune system of bees is therefore weakened him also.

"Pesticides weaken the colonies of bees and pathogens in benefit."[219] The GM plants can also have an impact on bees since plants emit themselves their own insecticide by genetic modification. The bees have never been in contact with the toxin of this soil bacterium used in this process. Either the bees have undergone a mutation at the result of this contact, either they do

133

not recognize the genetically modified plants as natural and avoid, either they are trapped and are poisoning by them.

"As well, after butiné sunflowers treated by neurotoxic pesticides, bees have abnormal behaviors, they are taken of seizures."[220] of children with autism are also of epileptic seizures. I myself have been witness to this poisoning of our pollinating if valuable and essential to our survival. I was sitting in the sidecar of a motorcycle, that of my husband, and we revert to a visit with friends in the Montérégie. A bee falls on the seat next to me. On the back, it turned on itself: what makes me think now to the behavior of children with autism when they rotate on themselves too. It flies in a spiral, and Drops. It raises and it is the wiper head with its legs vigorously, which resembles the flapping, behavior observed in children with autism. It tries to fly again, but it only succeeds in turn on itself by not reaching there on only a few centimeters away, and always in a spiral, what makes me think about the difficulty of children to walk. It arises on the edge and rubs again the head. Then, it falls in the bottom of the side-car on the back, the legs in the air, the abdomen curved. I looked around us and everything that I saw it was fields of Transgenic Maize in profusion. Farewell, my little bee! Despite his agony, I could not give him the coup de grace. The following day, I found dead there at the same place where I view the standby. In Quebec, it is the corn that receives the most pesticides, most of which is intended for the feeding of animals for slaughter.

Poor beasts!

"Corn Fed chemically treaty, beef is in head to its greater concentration of residues of pesticides, compared to any other food sold in the United States. It is also the meat most consumed by North Americans."[221] Approximately 90 per cent of the production of corn and oats will to livestock instead to counter the famine in the poor countries. When the pesticides are stored in living organisms, it is a bioaccumulation.

When animals eat plants that have been sprayed with these types of products, their organs and tissues become impregnated. When other animals eat these contaminated animals, toxic substances date back slowly the food chain and it is to the Summit of the latter that we find the greatest concentrations of pesticides and herbicides. The man is not immune to this pollution and ends by consumption of meat, fish and water containing pollutants.[222]

The use too abundant of pesticides contaminating everything that there is along the food chain. Wild animals are directly killed by pesticides. As we have seen, they also destroy the insects and parasites beneficial which otherwise neutralize insects and pests harmful, but instead, their destruction allows the proliferation of destructive insects, what the producers believe to be a resistance to the product.

At the time of their distress and their suffering in their passage to the slaughterhouse, their OS would release the toxins stored in their flesh, which could ensure that it oxidizes more rapidly forcing us to find ways for the alternative retain longer and give him a beautiful appearance.

Consume too much of animal protein can cause health problems. Traces of pesticides have been found in the fat of animals that we consume including those in red flesh. Among the animal fats are also the milk and egg yolks.

"The dairy products, fish and animal fat accumulate organochlorines (PCBS) because they coalesce in preference to fats; hormones, tranquilizers, vaccines, pollution abatement residues and pesticides are also found in animal flesh."[223]

The White Gold

Eggs and dairy products may interfere with the absorption of iron. The iron is important for the concentration. It is essential to the transportation of oxygen to the tissues and cells.

"The American Pediatric Academy has recently advised to refrain from feeding the new-born in the milk of cow, believing that this power was causing deficiencies in iron."[224] We know that iron deficiency may be caused also by the intolerance to gluten which abyss intestinal villi,. The rate of iron can be cancel in the presence too large of calcium. Therefore, the milk cow abîmerait also the intestinal mucosa?! The iron found in red meat oxyderait cholesterol, which in return could cause of disorders in the brain.

"Osteoporosis is not due to an inadequate intake of calcium in the power supply, but to various factors which prevent its assimilation or who facilitate its rejection."[225] The excessive use of solar cream could also contribute to osteoporosis. The milk does not contain vitamin D; that is why it would be added. Too much vitamin D in this form of supplement could be harmful in the long term for the intestines. We need the sunlight to synthesize Vitamin D, the true, which in turn helps to metabolize the absorption of calcium.

The milk would not be such a good source of calcium contrary to what one would believe. There is the calcium in several vegetables. The animals do not drink milk throughout their life. Why do they not have problems with their OS nor with their teeth as we?

135

Because their source in procurement in calcium is appropriate to their metabolism, which is not our case. The plants contain calcium in a form much more easily assimilated by our body. Our great consumption in dairy products ensures that we give less space to fruit and vegetables in a power supply which would be more balanced.

The milk of cow could have a link with the diabetes among children. More and more dairy cows are carriers of the virus bovine leukemia, a virus that is transmitted to humans and that resists even to the pasteurization. Is this just a coincidence if, of our days, the highest rate of leukemia is found among children aged 3 to 13 years, those who consume the most milk and who eat red meat?[226]

Some of the contamination to lead in some dairy products could come from crops along the road. On the road of the food poisoning, we can meet the beef of the Americans, the Quebec corn and potatoes in the Maritimes. Potatoes from the east of the country would receive up to 20 applications of pesticides. Despite all the warnings, the Canadian government has allowed this practice.

A small glass of arsenic with it?

In addition, the bottles of wine contain heavy metals dangerous for health. Approximately 20% of agricultural pesticides used in Europe are intended for vines. Of pesticide residues may therefore contaminate the wine. Several pesticides contain heavy metals. The seeds are treated with a pesticide containing mercury. Heavy metals including compounds in arsenic have been used as insecticides. Some herbicides and insecticides would contain arsenic. Several children with autism, including those of farmers, are intoxicated to the arsenic. Inorganic pesticides contain arsenic, of sulphate of copper, lead and mercury. It is found of arsenate of lead in some of these products as well as of the oxide of arsenite. Traces of arsenic have been found on insects as well as in the blood of birds causing a loss of feathers at the latter as well as mortality. The dangerousness of the pesticides on the basis of arsenic was discovered only after its use, so after that the marketing has been permitted.

Fungicides also contain heavy metals such as arsenic, even that of algaecides used as shock treatment for the water of the swimming pools. Arsenic is yet a deadly poison. Despite this, it aspergerait our cereals and fruit and vegetables with this product, as well as the food to feed animals, which in turn can contaminate the meat. Even the cigarette smoke would contain cadmium and arsenic from without doubt of this with what the tobacco plants have been treated. Traces of lead and cadmium have been found to the roots and in the leaves of some plants, including spinach.

"The soils which are regularly applied the manure of pigs and poultry can accumulate large quantities of heavy metals, capable to their turn to contaminate crops and constitute a threat to human health."[227] The chemicals are at the peak of the environmental hypersensitivity. The hidden toxins from our style of modern life are poisons. We are the victims of a internal pollution through the food, water and air. There would even be of lead and arsenic in some fertilizer. Fertilizer allow the plants to no longer need to feed themselves in depth.

"Plants thus processed do not set that 10% of fertilizer, 90% disperse in the environment."[228] The nitrates come from chemical fertilizers; they contribute to the pollution of water courses with a proliferation of algae reducing the intake of oxygen to other aquatic species.

The heavy metals, dioxins, furans, PCBS, pesticides accumulate in the body. They can harm the fetus and be found in breast milk.

The monoculture creates ideal sites for insects and weeds , thus creating a resistance to pesticides, which would require to use products more toxic, more pollutants and in larger quantities. The rotation of crops would allow a minimal use of these hazardous products.

"The current pollution of groundwater comes from 20 to 30 years of fertilizer application. Even if it stopped today to fertilize the soil, it would have to wait several decades before returning to a normal situation."[229] The DTT and organochlorines are still found in the flesh of fish and in the sediments in the course of water even if their use is prohibited in Canada since 20 years.

The water is the basis of the beginning of life on earth. The pollute destroys the basis even of life. A tiny part of pesticides reaches its target, the rest is garbage and accumulates in the environment.

The use of pesticides is 30 times more important than in 1942. There are approximately 70 000 products marketed in the form of herbicides, fungicides and insecticides, which is equivalent to 24 million tonnes annually. With the percolation of water, products used in the agricultural fields such as fertilizers, fertilizers and pesticides end up in the course of the water. This destroys as well the aquatic balance and reveals new phenomena, including the blue-green algae.

It is the excessive use of fertilizers that fact push more algae in the water, which causes damage to the marine ecosystem. The aquatic environment is deteriorating and it is any its flora and all its wildlife who suffer. Nitrates which are found in the water kill several aquatic species including fish, which are at the base of the food chain. Even the manure and slurry of liquid manure gather in the water, what destroy all the middle of aquatic life.

"In Canada, agricultural activities are at the origin of 80% of the marine pollution."[230] The presence of bad algae indicates a poor quality of the water. The phosphate would cause the disproportionate growth of aquatic plants, which depletes the water course in oxygen which otherwise would be more available to other species. The decline of the oxygen in the water is also due to an organic contamination from agriculture, municipal sewers as well as the intensive livestock.

Blue-green algae would be formed of aquatic microorganisms of the bacterial type and their proliferation could come from a bacterial resistance caused by the massive use of antibiotics in animal husbandry. People have suffered from neuromuscular disorders after eating shellfish that have fed of these algae. Of the dogs are become paralyzed after s be bathed in these waters. High levels of pesticides and chemical fertilizers have been found in oysters. "The Blue-green algae kill a large number of animal species terrestrial who drink these waters; a large number of fish, many plants."[231]

Modern agriculture is, with the use of sun creams, responsible in part for the destruction of corals. If the Solar cream can destroy the coral, imagine the difficulty that she can do to us. Industrial wastewater are doing their part in the aquatic pollution. The use of chlorine also decreases the oxygen in the water.

The contaminants found in water include chlorine, herbicides, insecticides, solvents, lead and arsenic. The nitrate, a chemical carcinogen found in the groundwater by the runoff of fertilizers, are not tolerated by infants and an exposure can cause the blue baby syndrome - which is often deadly. Atrazine is a herbicide which contaminates many reserves of water by the world and which has been linked to breast cancer and uterine coils in rats.[232]

Chemical fertilizers allow a large agricultural performance to the detriment of nutrient values natural, and are responsible for the massive pollution of water and soil. Thousands of tonnes of fertilizer are used each year. We no longer live in harmony with nature, exhausted soils are a food nutrient poor which weaken the organization of several living beings.

The earth is dying

"A soil devoid of microorganisms cannot fulfill its role of nurturing mother and becomes unfit for culture."[233] The bacteria in the soil help the roots to absorb the nutrients that the plant has need. If the organisms die, it will be necessary to use even more of fertilizer. The intensive culture induces a poverty of the soil.

"To increase their harvests, farmers use more and more fertilizers, pesticides and water. Chemical fertilizers make the soil more compact and more vulnerable to drought and to erosion."[234] The death of land fact drop the yield of crops to the hectare, which could eventually lead to a world hunger. The chemical substances accumulate in the soil and they may not deteriorate since these products have destroyed the microorganisms that had this function. The degradation of the soil has to consequences the erosion, leaching of the surface layer rich in minerals, landslides and the muddy waters of the rivers. The courses of water acidify not only because of acid rain, but also because of all that is spilled.

Incinerators of municipal garbage and industrial waste deposit of dioxin in the environment. Of harmful particles also travel in the air and deposited in the neighborhood and on nontarget plants that are consumed by animals also non-targeted.

The acidification of soil increases the bioavailability of heavy metals it contains. The pH of the soil influence of many microbial life just as the pH of our body. In return, a pH less alkaline in our body makes heavy metals even more toxic. The same goes for the soil.

The pollution of the waters of swimming pools

Although the chlorine used to disinfect contaminated water, it also contains harmful properties. It irritates the eyes, the skin and dehydrates the hair. Some chloroform vapor, a disinfectant substance behind in the form of a toxic gas irritant, would escape from the chlorinated water of the swimming pools and bathers are exposed. Among the symptoms found after prolonged exposure, there is memory loss, fatigue, voice difficulties, headache and sore throat, eczema, inflammation of the nasal passages, as well as problems of fertility and of disorders of sensitivities of pulmonary and cardiac. Of the chloroform would have been found in the blood plasma of bathers. It can contribute to the deficiencies of the liver and kidneys, organs that are extremely important in the detoxification.

"Epidemiological research shows that there is a relationship between the exposure of the skin to chlorinated organic substances and cancer of the skin. A lot of professional swimmers suffer from asthma."[235]

The Chlorine mixed with the aluminum of the sun creams would not good household with the skin. A cancer of the liver may even booting if the chlorinated water is swallowed frequently. It is the same on the drinking water of large cities treated with chlorine. As a result of this regular consumption and long-term, a cancer of the bladder, of fetal anomalies and abortions may occur. More there are swimming pools in a region, more people and, especially, children suffer from asthma. Babies who are going in the swimming pools of which the water is treated with chlorine are suffering more than other children of bronchiolitis. Exposure to chlorine has repercussions in the short and long terms. The doses of chlorine for swimming pools that are not respected can even lead to death. Chlorine is a corrosive product and oxidant. It is used in the power supply as a money launderer for bread more white than white and to launder the small raw carrots not organic. Just as the fluorine, chlorine could cause dental problems and to facilitate the release of mercury from dental amalgam in the body of humans.

Poisoning The existence

Pcbs, pesticides, arsenic, mercury, solvents and the plastic would act on the hormones including estrogen amending the sexual orientations. This would explain why there would be a lot more mortality at birth among baby boys and that this could have an impact also on the increasingly large number of children with autism in boys. Some animals would be came to the world with atrophied penis.

The chromated copper and other derivatives of copper in pesticides and herbicides could very well explain the blood poisoning of children with autism who have an unusually high rate of copper in their blood compared to the ratio of zinc. The copper would be toxic to children with autism if there is present in large quantity, because their system is unable to metabolize.

"Sustained exposure of the fetus to certain pesticides could significantly increase the risk of autism."[236] Organochlorines affect the operation of the neurotransmitters GABA and on the rate of hormone. Another form of intoxication can affect us, it is the genetic pollution. The seeds of genetically modified organisms can disperse their foreign genes and contaminate other species. It would be too early to assert that there is no danger to health in the

140

short, medium and long terms, as well as on the generations to come.

It took many years for the toxicity of some of these products is recognized and that they are finally banned in 1972. In the meantime, more than three million tonnes of this hazardous product have been widespread in the environment. In 1980, the World Health Organization (WHO) stated that, each year, pesticides were causing nearly twenty thousand deaths and almost three million poisonings various. Pcbs are spreading in the terrestrial and marine environment and affect the immune defenses and the reproductive organs of living organisms.[237]

The safety standards are calculated on only one product at a time by report to the average weight of an adult not considering the interaction of products between them or the weight of the babies. The limit of food poisoning say "acceptable" would be assessed according to the quantity that can be ingested daily during its entire existence without damage to health. The tolerable daily intake is not concerned of individual differences and does not consider the difficulties in some individuals to detoxify. Levels greater than the limit have been found on 10 residues of pesticides. The use of pesticides and fertilizers is executed in a manner very irrational. Their decomposition by the sun, the water and the microorganisms makes these chemicals even more toxic. What study has thought to the impact of the products in contact with the different elements in the environment and the interaction of all these products between them?

Half of the fruit, vegetables and cereals consumed in France contain residues of pesticides. Several pesticides are carcinogenic, affect the immune defenses or slowing down the growth of children. And the Department of Agriculture counterpart without batting an eyelash such products hazardous to health? The various departments of agriculture have had for a long time more likely to support intensive agriculture and highly productive than to worry about the health of consumers. This is due in part to the pressure from powerful agri-food lobbies.[238]

We are désinformés and manipulated. It should when not even die in ignorance. Of the poisonings took place in Iraq in 1972 by seeds treated with pesticides organomercuriels.

The manner in which the hazardous products are stored and transported may represent a risk to the environment and health, because of accidents, for example of the leaks, can occur. Some products defended in a certain place or country are simply sold where they are allowed or where monitoring is reduced if there is. With all exports and imports of foods, it can no longer be certain of the quantity of products which has been used to treat them. The regulation of other countries is different and less severe. In addition, despite the regulations in our own country, farmers are come their products elsewhere by Internet or by other processes. The regulation and monitoring of the use of these toxic products differ from region to region and from one country to the other. Other farmers will use a product intended for a plant to another plant. Several do not comply with the regulations.

People are sick every time they eat fruits or vegetables from other countries, probably because of the substances with which they have been sprayed. Since we eat Bio to the House, with fruits and vegetables the premises, all the family is better. However, there is nothing that is completely biological because the neighboring fields contaminate the other. Everything that can be done is to try to eat the most biologically possible, for example by making its own garden. Once again, attention must be paid to the seeds that you buy and the land that it is come.

What a beautiful invention!

Someone said to me with enthusiasm (and deep conviction) that pesticides are one of the most beautiful inventions of man, because in addition to having created jobs, it would have allowed to overcome hunger in the world. If this was the case, there would be more children die of hunger in the under-developed countries, whereas in Canada there are still children who do not eat to their hunger and who go to school without even having breakfast in the morning. Pesticides have not helped to curb poverty; on the contrary, they have contributed to increase the wealth of the richest countries. This beautiful Great Invention destroyed the lives of several organizations and even the ours, because people who think only of themselves want steak in their base all days, and want their portfolio and their bank account well filled even if human beings around suffer. This is the "I, me and me" which account! The automobile is also a beautiful invention, and yet, it creates a lot of pollution and therefore of health problems. The neurotoxicity of the DEET does extends not just to insects such as mosquitoes and flies.

"A product present in many insect repellents creams, DEET, has an unexpected effect and dangerous on the nerve cells of mammals."[239] The DEET has already killed live fish in the water of the bathers. It is a myth to believe that the products applied to

142

the skin are not absorbed by the latter and that their toxic substance cannot join the internal organs. The skin of children absorbs more easily the chemical products in the environment.

Almost all the chemicals that are placed on the skin, in particular in liquid form, are finally absorbed and enter the blood. DEET (content in repellents to mosquitoes and flies) is known to cause neurological damage. The Duke University Medical Center has concluded by studies in the laboratory rat that the long-term use of DEET kills neurons of the brain.[240]

Do not use DEET with a solar screen, because it reduces its efficiency and obliges us to apply more, which increases the rate of toxicity.

Studies have shown that the DEET causes the death of brain cells and changes in behavior in the rat after a frequent use and prolonged. This exposure causes the death of the neurons in the regions of the brain that control muscle movements, learning, memory and concentration. However, a frequent use and long-term of the DEET, in particular in combination with other chemicals or medicines, could lead to deficits in the brain in vulnerable populations, in particular children.[241]

Intoxication to DEET is manifested by involuntary movements, convulsions, disorders of the Walk and a loss of muscle control, dizziness, a change in heart rate, irritation of the skin, an alteration of the mental state, hallucinations, agitation, irritability, aggressiveness, an increase of burrs, malformations, vomiting, upset stomach, nausea, irritation of the eyes, a lack of coordination and fine motor skills. DEET is found in the blood two hours after the exposure on the skin. Moreover, it is not just toxic to the nervous system of the man.

"In studies with animals, the DEET has been linked to many harmful health effects such as damage to the DNA, a false layer, of congenital anomalies, problems with sperm and testes as well as damage to the brain."[242]

The DEET can lead to coma and death. Since 1960, a dozen deaths have been attributed to exposure to DEET.

In this regard, my son does not tolerate the sun creams or repellents to mosquitoes. The last time that it has been used, the next day, autistic symptoms reappeared. We use the Citronella and a cream biological solar and natural. It was the same regarding the chlorine in swimming pools. Today, ours works in salt.

Chapter 12

The weight of heavy metals on our health

143

From birth, the immune system starts to produce antibodies to defend themselves against invaders. Breast milk provides him with a good part of antibodies, but this is not all: heavy metals can also be transmitted from mother to baby through the placenta, breast milk and even the infant milk formula.

Throughout his life, the body does not cease to fight of substances that are harmful to its proper functioning and which can be harmful also for its normal development. Small doses are additive and accumulate. The mechanisms of defense would be overloaded with work, they would not to manufacture all the equipment of which the Organization has need. The degrees of toxicity of a child are seven times higher than those of an adult. The body of the smaller in growth and training is more likely to be intoxicated by heavy metals. They have more difficulty in eliminating environmental toxins. Person does not measure the quantity already established of heavy metals to the inside of the body of a child before him to make other. Inject a vaccine which contains heavy metals in the first minutes of his birth is harmful. The nervous system of children is in the course of development. It is therefore more vulnerable to exposure to pollutants such as heavy metals, and the brain is the part of the body are the most vulnerable to the intoxication to heavy metals. The brain of the autistic children would contain more heavy metals than that of other children.

In the person with autism, the natural ability of detoxification of the Organization in the face of heavy metals would be reduced and there could be a causal relationship (direct or indirect) between the exposure of the brain to heavy metals and some symptoms of autism. The toxicity of metals to the brain could explain, at least in part, the response of the brain decreased.[243]

More and more pupils in primary school are non-verbal cues and heavy metals to interfere in the development of the language. They decrease the intellectual quotient. The accumulation in the tissues as a result of low exposures becomes a chronic toxicity. Even rejected in small quantities, heavy metals are of micropollutants including their toxicity expands by bioaccumulation. The environmental causes explain the high rate of children with autism in the most industrialized countries. The symptoms of intoxication to heavy metals are strangely similar to those of autism, what you can see a little further by yourself.

The capabilities of children are affected by food in the first place which, even once washed, still contain these famous residues of pesticides. Traces of organophosphorus insecticides have been found in analyzes of taken blood from children.

In Canada, the source of arsenic would come from the power supply. The arsenic, under its inorganic form, would come in the composition of certain pesticides intended for agricultural activities such as those of the potato and cotton, as well as the orchards, same as in the storage of our food. "Lead arsenate,, doubly toxic, is a current employment to combat the Colorado potato beetle."[244]

Poisoning The more severe to the arsenic would be those that would have taken place accidentally when persons would be entered into contact with pesticides (insecticides, herbicides, fungicides) which contained of arsenate. A study would have been abandoned in 2008 because of the risks on the health of human guinea pigs volunteers.

By using on a long period of chemical compounds to protect the plants, the agri-food industry has led to the increase in the rate of lead, cadmium, mercury and copper in our soils formerly culturable, thus contaminating our food as well as the water. In addition, all of the tools of construction containing traces of solvents, paints, glues, paint removers which have been washed after use carry with them heavy metals in the course of water thus destroying the flora and the fauna. Most of these products are not biodegradable. Even the immune functions of the fish would be weakened or disrupted because of the fishermen would have caught fish with cancer and others with a reduced development of the brain. After having invaded the water, the soil and the air, heavy metals accumulate in all organizations of the living beings in a manner extremely dangerous. They threaten the survival of several plant and animal species while unbalancing Several ecosystems in nature. The contamination of the soil can cause adverse effects on the balance of ecosystems and on the food chain. The heavy metals do not degrade and accumulate in the food chain.

The reproductive capacity of the Man and the woman depends on a complex balance between different metabolic functions. External factors such as stress, increased pollution of the Environment (pesticides, solvents, heavy metals, hormones, etc.) and changes the mode of life (food, alcohol, smoking, etc.) appear to exert an influence more negative on fertility that what would admit commonly. The toxic metals (including heavy metals) are likely to fundamentally alter hormone metabolism as well as the fertility.[245]

There would, in the past few years, a decline of schoolchildren in primary, to the point that of regular teachers are move to other sectors of education. "Currently, it is estimated that in the industrialized countries, a man produces two times less of sperm that his grandfather was producing at the same age."[246]

Everything that is composed of plastic would also contain heavy metals or has already content very recently. Plastic crates and plastic pallets in would contain with high levels that exceed the permitted limits. The phthalates, a chemical product that consist some plastic objects, would be just as toxic as the bisphenol A. Most of these products may cause lesions to the organs including the brain. The accumulation of heavy metals causes the dementia and depression, even that of sleep disorders and the loss of the cognitive faculties. It is known that the intoxication to heavy metals can cause inflammations, then of chronic diseases (chronic fatigue syndrome, fibromyalgia, autism, hyperactivity) and even lead to neurodegenerative diseases (multiple sclerosis, Alzheimer and Parkinson diseases)."[247]

The hyperactivity is associated with peptides from the gluten and casein which their digestive enzymes have been destroyed by heavy metals. Personality disorders limit and the obsessive-compulsive disorders (OCD) who are treated and regarded as psychiatric illnesses could be in fact that a poisoning to opiates by reason of intoxication to heavy metals. They would also be responsible behavior disorders because of this poisoning to the peptides opiates which act as of morphine on the neurotransmitters. The gluten and casein prevent the maturation of the brain. Opioid substances saturate the brain and inhibit the social links as the downturn on itself, the indifference and the absence of the language. They would be the cause of violence among young people and in society in general. They are also devastating to the functioning of the thyroid gland.

"Traces of pesticides affect the hormonal production of the thyroid, causing a hypersensitivity to chemicals and can cause an increase in irritability and aggressiveness."[248] diseases following modern are in effect created by the man: conduct disorder, hyperactivity, depression, dyslexia, school failure, attention deficit and difficulties to concentrate. The toxic immune syndrome would become the illness of the industrial era. It cause several serious health problems. The environmental poisons act as small time bombs.

The heavy metals disrupt the functioning of our vital organs. Among the catalysts of oxidation are found the lack of oxygen, the overconsumption of junk food, solvents, heavy metals, glues, pesticides and herbicides, because they make our body acid. If the pH of our body is too acid, heavy metals will be more difficult to dislodged. Therefore, a field compromises acid detoxification, that is why it is necessary to favor alkali foods including dairy products and gluten are not part. Consume too much of these foods prevents our body to clean properly. On the one hand, heavy metals, destroy the digestive enzymes of these two proteins that we no longer to absorb and metabolize, on the other, eat prevents the heavy metals out. This is another vicious circle to the benefits of pollutants.

The essential minerals are antagonists of heavy metals, but these, causing digestive disorders, prevent the absorption of minerals, then these become inactive and therefore cannot combat the intoxication. As well, the heavy metals emit and take the place of essential minerals themselves, who in turn, may not fulfill their function which is to combat them. For example, of lead and cadmium can take the place of the calcium and upset as well the biochemical reactions of the body and the enzyme system.

A low rate in selenium, an essential mineral for detoxification, would result from a poor diet or a difficulty in the absorption of nutrients, contacts with toxic heavy metals: chemical solvents, pesticides and herbicides. The Selenium, in addition to be absolutely essential to the maintenance of certain enzymes related to digestion, also has the function of an antioxidant. This essential mineral can also enable, set and facilitate the extraction of heavy metals. The deficit in selenium would be responsible for a lower immune reaction. Here is another example which shows that the heavy metals hamper the functioning of the immune system. The lack of selenium would increase the inflammatory response, which may cause allergic reactions to certain foods or substances. All this can lead to degeneration and to a delay in growth or to a pervasive development disorder.

A level too low in potassium would also indicate a weakness in the enzymatic functions as well as a nutritional imbalance. It is a disorder gastro-intestinal tract caused also by the intoxication to heavy metals which could cause this deficit in potassium. The diarrhea would eliminate therefore a good quantity of essential elements. The reaction of certain enzymes would depend on the rate of minerals which some would act as a catalyst. The low concentration of manganese would come, as the other essential minerals, a bad food absorption and a bad functioning of the digestive system. It is the same regarding the level low in boron in several children with autism. The poor absorption creates a nutrient deficit enabled by the lack of enzymes. This deficit causes a decrease in the physical endurance as well as fatigue. A risk of infertility and a loss of weight to the birth have been noticed in some cases. There is more and more infertile couples and advanced age is not always the case.

Heavy metals can seep into the Semen and cause a mutation of the DNA to the offspring. "What are the pollutants, heavy metals and other toxins which, when they have penetrated the body, go to the interior of the cells to the contact of the DNA that they are mutate."[249] The industrial pollution, including that to toxic metals can cause genetic mutations and thus bring changes to the functioning of the immune system. Heavy metals can cause bone lesions, neurological disorders, genetic mutations and cancers. They destroy the biology of living cells and disrupt the biochemical balance.

The Mercury (or other metals) could inhibit the antioxidant functions and détoxicantes of glutathione. Laboratory mice susceptible to autoimmune diseases, exposed to repeated injections of thimerosal, show signs of damage neurological and behavioral as well as a oxidative stress increased, correlatively to a fall in the rate of intracellular glutathione.[250]

The heavy metals prevent the production of energy in the cells by blocking the enzymatic repair of DNA. This can lead to the mitochondrial disease. They can enter the body in various ways such as by respiration, the power supply and the absorption through the pores of the skin. If the organization does not happen to get rid of properly, a buildup occurs in the tissues. This makes the poison, this is not just the quantity, but the time where occur the poisoning and the increase of the toxicity with the contact of the other products.

Mercury, Arsenic, lead and cadmium are recognized as the heavy metals the most toxic. They can cause pathological disorders, physiological, as well as metabolic disorders that can inhibit the operation of the immune system; this defect is at the base of the autistic disorders. The heavy metals would play a major role in the onset of autism. There is a close link between a poisoning to heavy metals and various immune disorders, neurological and intestinal disorders. Poisoning to mercury, cadmium, lead, arsenic, tin and aluminum would be those that contribute the most. Most of the autistic children are intoxicated to one or several of these toxic

148

metals, but to varying degrees; the most common are those to mercury, lead, arsenic and cadmium.

The toxins that can cause of neurological disorders would go through the liver which is responsible for the filter if it works well, and are then evacuated by the intestines If those are also in good health, which is rarely the case in autistic children. They adhere to the intestinal membrane and can cross it. After having travelled in the body, certain molecules then return to the intestines that they damage more. They would undermine the new immune system then recross the membrane and travel again in the blood by creating other damage. Another vicious circle installs and persists as well. The toxins are circulating in the blood and cause various disorders including a brain dysfunction. The heavy metals that are circulating in the blood can damage the bodies and may even be the cause of development carcinogenic. If this is the case, the vaccines could therefore be one of the causes for which the rate of cancer is on the rise. The Autism is an autoimmune disease like cancer: In both cases, it is a disorder immune. For example, the kind of antibody which should have the highest rate is the one that has the least, and vice versa. This would also explain the adverse reactions to vaccines.

A delay in the development of general and of verbal failures are the first signs of intoxication to heavy metals observed in a child with a tendency toward the autism; this would also explain the regression on the plan of the language to be the result of one or several vaccines. There is more and more children who are dysphasic or who have a delay of the language with speech difficulties, or who have completely lost the vocabulary words already acquired. The mercury poisoning because of difficulties of pronunciation. Among the other signs of poisoning in the rest of the population, we find: chronic fatigue, the feeling of not being well in his skin, depression, chronic diseases in expansion such as cancer and diabetes, as well as the irritability, aggressiveness and self-mutilation.

The whole world is intoxicated with one or several metals without even the knowledge and to different degrees, especially if one feels one of these diseases or one of these Associated symptoms: depression, diabetes, allergies, muscle pain, migraines, insomnia, fatigue, frequent sinusitis, mycosis, vertigo, burns, ulcers, metallic taste in the mouth, contraction of the muscles including or not involuntary movements, tingling in the legs, digestive disorders, nervous problems, difficulties to concentrate.

If the Depression and the self-inflicted injury are caused by the mercury and not of other heavy metals, then vaccines and some drugs could well also be responsible for the increase in the rate of suicide. This scourge is more and more common in modern history and which affects more and more young people, even that of the workers who are often in contact with these toxic products. Vaccines and Drugs would become an evil of society, then that they have been designed to combat the evil.

The Arsenic

The arsenic would be a violent poison and toxic. It is a hazardous heavy metal even at low doses. If the subject is exposed to several occasions, even if it is taken in small quantities on a certain period, the effects can be devastating. Napoleon Bonaparte would have been poisoned by arsenic.

The arsenic, after having travelled in the blood, would normally be eliminated through the urine and by the sweat. The Baths very hot or saunas can help the detoxification. The ability of detoxification differs from one person to another, especially if the accumulation of toxins has caused the anomalies to the defense mechanisms become unable to clean the body properly. Heavy metals are attacking the system that has the function to eliminate them. Arsenic could accumulate in the digestive system and cause diarrhea. Normally, small quantities can be excreted by tracks the liquids from the body. Intoxication in the long term, as indicated in the analysis of hair, would affect the nervous system. In addition, it would destroy also the essential minerals which feed the digestive enzymes. Therefore, it could be a trigger of food allergies including those related to the peptides that lead to autistic symptoms. The arsenic would be the rival of the selenium, an important mineral to maintain the immune system in good health. It is necessary to increase the essential minerals of the body in order to better combat the heavy metals.

The nervous system is the most vulnerable to the toxicity of hazardous products such as heavy metals that have an impact on the dementia, the mood, the loss of the cognitive faculties, memory loss and sleep disorders. Arsenic does not cause just damage to the nervous system, but also to the liver, lungs and intestines. It can cause abdominal pain, nails fragile, stomach disorders and digestive, convulsions, drowsiness, hair loss, headache, cancer of the liver and lungs, muscle pain, muscle spasms, irritability, extreme fatigue, respiratory diseases and swallowing difficulties.

According to some researchers, a very low level would have beneficial effects in the body, but we do not know at what dose and at what level since the results were derived from experiments on rats as if our system resembled that of rodents. And yet, which is controversial in this study is that rodenticides, i.e. the poisons to rats, contain arsenic. A high percentage in the food and water could also prove fatal.

Arsenic can cause damage and lead to complications in various systems: digestive, intestinal tract, enzymatic, nervous, circulatory, as well as a poor functioning immune. Among the consequences of such intoxication, there would be opportunities to develop cancer, damage to the brain and the intestines including an acute gastrointestinal that can cause very serious abdominal disorders, diarrhea, nausea and vomiting, as well as problems to the bodies which an anomaly in the liver by an alteration of enzymatic functions, without forgetting a destruction of blood vessels responsible of the immunity and the transport of oxygen due to a deceleration of the activities of the red and white cells. The intoxication to arsenic could lead to a chromosomal alteration thus changing the genetic material leading to an inability to reproduce or to a reproductive incompatibility. This mutation triggers of disorders in several systems of the body.

An exhibition in the short, medium and long terms to this toxic heavy metal could cause numbness at the end of Members, redness and skin rashes, tingling, losses of reactions drive, a deterioration of sensory responses, poor fetal formations, neurological disorders, muscle weakness and a decrease in the Speed sensorial. Do you not of symptoms related to autism? Several children with autism intoxicated to the arsenic have digestive disorders and heart. The decrease in red blood cells and white led the cells to a lack of oxygen and nutrients. The arsenic therefore cause damage to blood vessels. It irritates the lungs making them more vulnerable to infections and would be responsible for a part of the cancer of the skin.

Of the workers in the plantations of fruit would have suffered from brain damage after having used insecticides to arsenate. It was the cause of inflammations of the digestive tube, a excessive thirst and renal failure. The arsenic also cause dysfunctions of the thyroid gland. In general, heavy metals are endocrine disruptors which act on the hormonal balance of living species as well as on growth and development, behavior, reproduction and cellular energy. It causes irreversible effects on the fetus and children. This intoxication can be at the base of the precocious puberty, of testicular cancer, breast and prostate. Some heavy metals irritate the natural hormones and block the communication between the cells.

"The effects of endocrine disrupters can induce major health problems such as infertility, abnormal development of the fetus, the precocious puberty, cancers, diabetes, obesity, of neurological disorders, learning disabilities and many others."[251]

The drugs and the pollutants are blocking the activity of hormones and the functions of the bodies. The Infertility is a way that nature has established to protect the progeny to prevent that we put on the world of children poisoned, sick or disabled. When the toxic dose of arsenic is reached, is found in the brain causing of course of neurological disorders and nervous disorders Sensory and engines. This poison mainly located in the liver and kidneys and blocks their functions. It irritates the digestive tube, disrupts the nutrition in cells and tissues, blocks the enzymes, gives gastrointestinal disorders, muscle weaknesses, tingling in the extremities, brittle nails, a copious salivation, of motor disorders and walking, and causes cardiac arrhythmias. The arsenic increases the risk of cancer and type 2 diabetes.

Of genetic mutations have been observed in infants whose mothers had consumed water contaminated by arsenic in Thailand. Up to now, nobody suspected that genetic abnormalities could affect the progeny of the victims.

It has also been the cause of brain tumors and skin lesions. We cannot avoid exposures to arsenic since we find everywhere in the environment.

The foods represent the most significant route of exposure and the more common to organic arsenic, particularly crustaceans, meats, poultry, cereals and dairy products. In the past, household products such as paints, dyes, rodenticides and drugs against asthma and the psoriasis contained inorganic arsenic. These products are no longer commonly used.[252]

There is of the arsenic in wood preservatives, herbicides, glasses, pesticides, metal, meat and seafood, fungicides, Defoliants, desiccators, fertilizer, medicines, water, cigarette smoke, chemical industries. The air, water, soil, the treated wood and some electronic devices in contain; as well as the glass, the glass and crystal, and the latter may contain other metals such as lead and cadmium. The Chlorine, widely used for several years, is now considered that can be toxic, which has revealed the filters to the salt on the market, less harmful to our health.

"The food of animal origin, in particular the seafood, provide the largest proportion of arsenic from the power supply. Cereals and starchy foods such as rice and potatoes contain appreciable quantities of arsenic."[253] of cultures would be watered by the water would contain and which ends up pick up in the aquifers which feed our wells. Of the deposition of arsenic that there would also be in the soil would come from chemical fertilizers, defoliants and desiccants. Of the particles present on the leaves and on other plants could be ingested by animals whose flesh is successful in our plates. It seems that these products have been much used in the past and that their use would today be prohibited or tolerated only in certain regions and for certain crops, including those intended for the feeding of animals, up to the liquidation of the old stocks. But it remains no less that even if it is used less and less, as some claim, the soil remains contaminated because the arsenic does not degrade and accumulates. In 2002, arsenic acid would still have been authorized and used as a herbicide, insecticide and rodenticide in the United States that many of the food products consumed here in come from. Even fourmicides in contain. In places where the soils are sandy, water would cross more quickly the soil layers thus preventing the microorganisms to break down appropriately these toxic particles, which could pollute water courses and the groundwater resources.

"The industrial inputs agricultural and can multiply 10 to 20 times the amount of arsenic naturally contained in the soil."[254] In addition, still today, treatments for grass, golf courses, course of school, sports grounds would contain a derivative of arsenic. Of arsenate of calcium would have also been used in agriculture. The horses have already been contaminated with arsenic of herbicides used on the hay. Many agricultural soils have been contaminated by arsenic, which has been used as a herbicide and insecticide. It is not biodegradable. Copper Arsenate would already have been used in the dyes to candies, as well as the colorful candy wrapped in paper tinted. The wine, beers and salads can contain. There would be in the paper also painted. Of the radishes and beets in would contain. The blackening of roots and leaves of the plants is a sign of contamination of the soil. The arsenic would have been used on apples.

"Arsenic is always added to the animal food, particularly in the United States , as a method of prevention of the disease and on the stimulation of the growth."[255] Not surprising that we find the highest rate of children with autism in the United States.

The chromated copper is this green dye on the treated wood. Although a power pole green tinted either planted at a few meters of our artesian well, extensive analyzes of our water revealed the rates of heavy metals at the bottom of the standard. But which establishes this normality? This contamination to arsenic comes from somewhere. It is from the structures of wood playgrounds for children? It seems that the wood is more treaty of our days at the Arsenic, but it took them several years before to realize his dangerousness, and no study would have been made prior to the marketing of this process to know its toxicity.

Other research from governmental bodies have made me see that each belie what the other reveal. It is as if we were trying to we hide something. One day, I receive a press release informing me of the possible presence and the potential of arsenic in the fields of potatoes mainly from the maritime provinces, because it is a region where the there would be the highest rate of arsenic present in the sedimentary layers deep. In this region, we would have found the presence of this toxic product in the soil and water. A representative of the Ministry of Agriculture has yet responded that the pesticides on the basis of arsenic are no longer permits since long in the country. And yet, a member of my family by alliance is a Professor in agriculture in the Maritimes, precisely, and he told us the opposite. It has revealed to us that these are not just pesticides used in the Maritimes who would be on the basis of chromated, but also those used in Quebec and the other Canadian provinces. "The arsenic has been removed of pesticides for domestic use, but the commercial use of the imported arsenic remains high."[256]

If the potato grows in a contaminated soil to arsenic and if it receives in addition of pesticides to arsenic and water contaminated with this toxic metal, it is one more reason to buy food bios and premises. In addition, some potatoes would be covered with another chemical to prevent to germinate.

If is found of heavy metals in the Poisons intended to get rid of certain harmful animals whose rodenticides, the fact to find in fertilizer, fertilizer and pesticides which affect our food could in principle we also poison since we were often compared to these bugs in laboratory tests. The products of tangible hygiene would contain almost all of the heavy metals in order to preserve of bacteria and fungi, and these products can be absorbed by the skin, such as Shampoos that contain arsenic, the lead in the makeup and a derivative of the mercury in the mascara. But why these products are they still on the market? Of household cleaners and industrial also contain, especially among the disinfectants. The antibacterial disinfectants for the hands would destroy the natural flora of our hands which combat by themselves the bacteria that we are so afraid. In addition, this product dries the skin. One day, while we were visiting my parents, our children have taken a bath and their grand-mother has used its own products. To return to the House, our son has seen reappear of autistic symptoms.

The tin

The tin is part of the toxic heavy metals. It is there in pesticides, but also in the glass industry, ceramics, and plastic. We would have the tin in the alloy and the welds in the lead pipes for copper from old houses and old water systems that supply water to the schools in the large urban centers. These pipes of old houses would be made of an alloy composed at the time of lead and tin, since it is a white metal which lends itself easily to the Welding and which is resistant to corrosion; it enters in the composition of various alloys such as copper, lead, nickel and zinc. It would have been also used in mixtures of silverware. The soil and the air could contain as well as the cosmetics, dental amalgam, the welds of certain cans of food and drinks. "Of metal sheets coated with tin are used for the manufacture of cans, containers for aerosols and equipment of dairy."[257]

Can be found in the form of chloride of tin. It is a metal that is often used in the medical field despite its toxicity. "There is something fishy!" The fluoride in would also contain, which could damage the enamel of the teeth. Surprising that wild animals have not decay. New toothpastes are placed on the market without fluorine for the people who really want to keep their teeth longer without poisoning and while preserving a better health. Fluorine would transform the amalgam in a methylated form more toxic. Fluorine would trigger the genetic predisposition to allergies or would be an accomplice. Added to the water, it would increase the risk of cancer. "The administration of fluorine to children would have resulted in a decrease of the capacity of the brain, the motor restlessness, anemia, thinning hair and especially considerable unrest of the immune defenses with, for consequences, recurrent respiratory infections and otitis media."[258]

Fluorine would also be used in agriculture in the herbicides, pesticides, fungicides and insecticides. This product is therefore highly toxic. It would also use to kill cockroaches and as poison to rats. High concentrations of organochlorine pesticides and expose children with ADHD.

Despite that he risk of contaminating our food, it is puts in the mouth to each brushing. In addition, the toothpaste would contain the aluminum because its containing could contaminate the content. It would be also used in drugs to increase their longevity as in of antibiotics, neuroleptics, anti-inflammatory, antihypertensives, tranquilizers, in surgery and for the sterilization of equipment. We would use in the power supply as a sweetener and for the fermentation of beer.

"The fluorine is a toxic gas very responsive and very dangerous to manipulate which, in contact with the skin, causes burns. Its extracts are used for nuclear energy, the manufacture of Teflon and insecticides."[259]

The fluoride added to the water would contain heavy metals, especially the one from China and which is used in municipal water supplies in the United States. Where to dump the waters fluorinated worn? Of sun creams contain fluorine to check its effect of fat. Fluorine would represent a danger for the degradation not only dental, but also skeletal. It may therefore be one of the Causes of osteoporosis. It may cause a delay of growth, of mental disorders and renal impairment. It would reduce the functions of the thyroid gland. Its toxicity by the oral route may have an impact on fertility. It could have mutagenic and carcinogenic. In general, fluorine would cause disturbances in liver, kidney, testes, thyroid gland, the skeleton and to the dentition. By the very fact, it would destroy the enamel of the teeth by its corrosive effect.

Phthalates are contained in the dishes and toys to children. It is difficult to know the content of toxic toys. Phthalates are toxic as well as the plastic. Of cosmetics by also contain especially as fixing agent. They can cause cancer of the testicles. They would cause anomalies male reproductive use by alteration of the development of the testis during pregnancy.

"A phthalate widespread causes after three days the disappearance of 40% of the germ cells in fetal."[260]

The manufacturers would not be obliged to indicate the toxicity of their products on the labels.

"An abnormal rate of phthalates that are toxic to the reproductive cells for men has been detected in some preparations for infants."[261]

The pénétrerait tin in the body by the pores of the skin, by the ingestion of contaminated food and by the respiration of the polluted air. Excessive exposure to tin would cause irritation to the eyes. Our son complained regularly of irritation in the eyes by rubbing them with two hands. The intoxication in the tin also causes damage gastrointestinal, muscle weakness, as well as anemia, which would explain the reason for which its rate of iron was so low. The tin would also be responsible for intestinal inflammation causing chronic The syndrome of the intestine porous, nausea, vomiting, diarrhea and colitis. Fluorine would also be responsible for the leaky gut. A destruction of enzymes that are responsible for the degradation of proteins follows. The enzymes would be inhibited, that is to say that their ability to react is slowed by the excess of the presence of heavy metals. The tin would also be responsible for frequent infections such as ear infections, colds, flu due to the weakening of the immune system. It also would cause problems to the engine system and disorders in the nervous system. Among the other symptoms, there is respiratory disorders including the cough without apparent cause and the shortness of breath to the slightest efforts. There are symptoms very similar if one compares those caused by intoxication to heavy metals with those that are apparent to autistic disorders.

In addition, tin can tackle the urinary system. It disrupts the growth. It may cause depressions, damage to the brain, of sleep disorders, anger, a deficiency of red blood cells, an alteration of the chromosomes, a immune dysfunction, damage to the liver. It would be another neurological toxicity. It disturbs the endocrine system and also causes skin irritations. It would be very toxic to the algae.

Lead

The lead, although it has been removed from the essence of the cars, would have been added in the toys for children. The lead is a heavy metal that has been used in the manufacture of paints for jewelry and some toys to children. It is a neurotoxic and has effects on the development of the brain. What happens to children who suck the mine of lead of their pencil?

Of the substances used in decoration in the world of construction represent a danger to health. In Europe, some paintings in vivid colors and some white pigmentation still contain lead, but in other forms and hidden under other names. If the rate of concentration does not exceed 0.15%, the manufacturer would not even be required to indicate on the label. Who would buy toys to children on which would be written on the packaging: "may contain lead, a toxic heavy metal that may be harmful to the physical and mental health of your child"?

"The formaldehyde (formalin) met sometimes in Synthetic Dyes for hair is a carcinogen by inhalation. Some hair dyes also contain lead, a heavy metal carcinogen."[262]

The old paint of old houses contained of the lead which the dust can be sucked especially during the renovations, which would have already led children to the paralysis and neurological disorders. Before 1950, the painting of houses in contained. Thus, exposed parents may have transmitted a sensitivity environmental chemical to their children. From 1950 to 1980, the paintings would have been composed still lead, but in less large quantities. The leaded paint would always be used in the staining of the plastic bags of groceries and stores, because some of these bags would come from China where the lead would still be allowed because their cost of production is minimal. How many people are also serve as these bags to cover food and as bags to lunch? Of toys manufactured in China would be more likely to contain lead to even their painting. The lead in toys would be responsible for transmissible and anemia.

The wooden toys - often sold for their green side - contain very often formaldehyde at high concentrations or heavy metals. Phthalates, formaldehyde or heavy metals are present in the composition of a number of dolls or teddy bears.[263]

The antibacterial products may contain mercury and lead. There may be lead in the glass, as well as lead and cadmium in the ceramic. We would have this heavy metal in the piping, tobacco smoke , welding, pesticides, Glazes with pottery, etc.

"If it is exposed to the heat or the rays of the sun and also, simply, by the process of aging, the PVC releases of lead in the form of a Dust that accumulates on the surface of the product."[264] To make the rigid PVC and sustainable, the industry would add of lead and cadmium. We would use for the manufacture of toys for children and of consumer products.

Even if the lead has been removed from the petrol since several years, it remains stored in the environment. In addition, Canadian industries would continue to reject in the air a volume of lead significantly higher than the U.S. average.

"As well, it was learned that the pollution by lead date of 3000 years and by the copper of 2500 years. Small consolation: our descendants will be able to track all the harm that we have inflicted on the land with our leading-edge technologies and all those to come."[265]

158

The game can be intoxicated to heavy metals. The presence of lead would have been found in the meat of cervids and corvids. We would have more pesticides in the meat of animals that are fed in cultivated fields. The hunters would have found of radioactive wild boar in the mountains after the Chernobyl disaster. In the rumen of a cow in France would have been found lead balls after she had consumed in corn fodder. The Silage with the lactic fermentation facilitates the impregnation of lead in plants, which would have been able to go up to contaminate the milk. The tobacco plants absorb heavy metals out of the soil yet more easily than the other. The kidneys of certain animals, even that their liver, would not be edible because of their content of pollutants such as heavy metals. This lead can be ingested by the man by the consumption of meat.

The lead balls of the guns which were used to shoot down the big game dispersed particles of lead in his flesh washed away by the blood during the last heart beat. The pigs would have suffered from lead poisoning when this meat would have been given to eat. Ammunition do not contain just the lead, but sometimes of mercury and cadmium. This are not all rifle bullets which reached their target, some falling in the nature on the ground and in the water, which has contaminated the environment. The lead can remain in the flesh of the animal which did not die and heal the wound, but another animal that feeds on them could become contaminated. The bullets of hunting that accumulate in the swamps can intoxicate wild geese and ducks. Wild animals can consume plants that contain residues of cartridges. The contamination of ecosystems would therefore be underestimated.

The birds contaminated with lead have their central nervous system affected. The birds found wounded or killed by the cars would have the accumulated lead in their OS, which would have slowed their reflex. The lead is disperse in the surrounding area by birds injured at the time of the impact.

The birds Victims of chronic intoxication or acute die and are consumed by scavengers or necrophagous insects, which in their turn, will contaminate those who will eat, etc. The animals weakened by the contamination are killed by predators or the man for their consumption. The whole of the food chain is reached with including animals of game type which can subsequently be consumed by the man.[266]

The lead because of neurobehavioral disorders, a intellectual deterioration, blocks the function of several enzymes, decreases the amount of red blood cells (anemia) and would be responsible

159

for a certain form of cancer. The lead would even be neurotoxic for bees endangered. Because of hunting, 1500 tons of lead would end up in the environment in Canada every year.

Lead affects the brain, retards the growth, because of the attention deficit disorder, learning, behavior problems and of development.

"The lead is a neurotoxic substance powerful often associated with nervous disorders and behavioral disorders including hyperactivity and attention deficit disorder."[267] lead because of the damage to the brain, the blood system and the liver. It reduces the intelligence and night at the mental development. This is not surprising that there are as many problems in the schools with a piping which contains lead. Damage to the nervous system by the lead have devastating effects on the behavior and the intellectual development.

"Various dyes and additives contained in the majority of lipsticks contain toxic heavy metals. Lead in particular is a metal that is harmful and carcinogenic which acts on the nervous system, the kidneys, the OS, the heart and the blood. It is a greater risk for pregnant women."[268] It also causes of growth disorders, muscle weakness, hallucinations and convulsions.

"The first signs of lead poisoning in are the problems of learning and behavior."[269] Why do not change the plumbing of the schools in the large urban centers, as well as their drinking water supply system!

Lead interferes with the biological functions normal and the Metabolic functions of base. It accumulates in the organs such as the liver, brain, heart and disrupts their functions. It decreases the renal capacities to evacuate the toxins. It may move the essential minerals. He is hunting minerals, including calcium, and takes its place by blocking the reaction of this mineral on enzymes. The enzyme activity is disrupted by the presence of heavy metals.

Here is particularly what we blame the lead: abdominal pain, allergies, anorexia, arthritis, autism, back pain, blindness, cardiovascular disorders, decrease of cartilage, disorders of coordination, constipation, deafness, depression, dyslexia, emotion, encephalitis, migraine, weakness, hypertension, a disorder of the thyroid gland, impotence, decreased immune and intellectual quotient, indigestion, infertility, insomnia, irritability, joint disorder, etc.

"These parasites can affect, among other things, the operation of neurological and muscular, the use of vitamins, energy level, the integrity of the intestinal wall and the use of hormones."[270] The phenol content in the fragrances can also cause of disorders in the central nervous system and the immune system. The mouthwash to ethanol and phenol would be toxic and carcinogenic, and could cause other disorders of health.

Atmospheric deposition of pollutants contribute to acid rain which alter the pH of the soil which, becoming more acid, help more heavy metals to install any as in our body. The pH less alkaline destroyed the living organisms of the soil as well as the useful bacteria to the inside of us.

The aluminum

It would of aluminum in the paper and the metal sheets, packaging of food, food animals, antacids, aspirins, exhaust gas of vehicles, yeasts, beer, bleached Flour, cans, ceramic, filter cigarette, color additives, construction materials, utensils and containers of kitchen, cosmetics, dental amalgam, deodorants, drinking water, dust, insulation of the wiring, medicines, dairy products, nasal spray, pesticides, pollution, soil, tobacco smoke, toothpaste, treated water, vanilla powder, baking powder, vaccines.

Lipstick, varnishes, bottom of complexion, creams of care, several of these products in direct and continual contact with our skin contain of the aluminum. A day of Solar cream to the beach would thus amount to spread on his skin, permeable, let us not forget, 1 g of aluminum. Its action could contribute to the aging of the epidermis and be linked to the incidence of cancer of the skin.[271]

The sun creams would transform solar energy into free radicals, they contain chemical substances Carcinogenic, which have an effect on estrogen and can damage the liver. The frequent use of solar filters would also lead to the risk of breast cancer and the decrease of the semen from the man. If it destroys corals, what can it we induce in wrong?

The aluminum would be also in dentifrices and bars of soap, cheese industry, the Foundry of ores, the water in the cities, food and beverages, canned, table salt, food additives. It can also be found in the breast milk of which many people preach the merits, often because of antiperspirants which contain. Just think that the aluminum can be absorbed by the pores of the skin and will make as well into the breast milk gives me the chills. In addition, the child, in tétant, can directly absorb since it can extend up to the nipple. Studies have shown a link between the use of antiperspirant to basis of aluminum and breast cancer in women.

A study published in 2003 by the European Journal of Cancer Prevention has found a correlation between the early diagnosis of

161

breast cancer and Antiperspirants-deodorants. In 2004 and 2005, the researcher Phil Darbre emits the hypothesis that specific substances in deodorants such as the Conservatives called parabens, or bolts as the aluminum chloride used in the antiperspirants can enter the bloodstream or accumulate in the breast tissue, where they contribute to strengthen or to imitate the effects of estrogen, which stimulates the growth of breast cancer cells.[272]

Applied on the skin of mice, traces of aluminum were found in the blood, urine, the brain and the placenta. The antiperspirant is a drug because it modifies the operation of a component: the skin. He formed the plugs, gelatinous in the ducts of the sweat glands. It is worse for the blocking of the pores of the skin if the antiperspirant is applied immediately after the shower when the pores are still open. The aluminum can remain stuck in the lymphatic glands.

Sweat is a natural way to evacuate the toxins like the fact to urinate. The saunas are recommended for the elimination of heavy metals. It is as if was used to a heavy metal to prevent the other metals of exit. Therefore, the use of antiperspirants prevents us not just sweating, but also prevents our body to clean, which overload the liver and kidneys of a additional work. The salts of aluminum tighten the pores of the skin, affecting the mechanism to exercise. This ensures that smells and toxins may not leave the body and become an aggression that can cause inflammatory reactions and damage the sweat glands. The toxins that may not leave the body through the sweat have no place to go; they store therefore in the tissues. There would be of the aluminum salt also in the products of care of the face, body scrubs, nail polish, makeup removers, and care products for the body. The accumulation of aluminum in the body as a result of the use of products that contain has been involved in the emergence of various pathologies such as Alzheimer's disease which would have increased with the massive use of antiperspirants. Only, the industry of these products is trying to deny the discoveries.

A man who would be allergic to the aluminum can not tolerate antiperspirants which contain; this puts me the chip to the ear concerning adverse reactions to some of the children who receive vaccines that contain. The aluminum could therefore be a trigger allergies. And allergies of parents should be considered as a factor that can trigger an adverse reaction in their child after receiving a vaccine.

It seems that the perspiration would not smell as such and that it is mainly the fermentation by bacteria and waste from which cause a smell. The know that one uses have a pH acid, which makes the ground more viable for these bacteria. To shave would be counter-indicated, because the hairs help to evacuate perspiration away from the skin. If there are hairs to this place, it is for a good reason that Dame Nature has placed there. In addition, most of these deodorants are made with a basis of alcohol, which stimulates the sweat forcing us to apply more. But what happens when the sweat is stimulated by the deodorant and that the Antiperspirant the blocks to the inside of the fabrics? It results in the accumulation of toxins in the cells, which can damage the DNA. If the aluminum is a neurotoxin that causes damage to the DNA is that it has a epigenetic effect that can cause cancer.

Antiperspirants to aluminum would be responsible for damage to nerves and autoimmune diseases. They would cause problems for lymphatic glands around the underarms. They also affect the endocrine system. And yet, we injects the aluminum with vaccines.

In spray or to ball, deodorants antiperspirants can contain up to 20% aluminum, which raises many questions, including the link between breast cancer and the aluminum. In 2007, British researchers have measured the aluminum content of breast tissue of 17 patients with cancer. The concentration was significantly higher in the region of the chest closest to the armpit.[273]

Individuals with impaired renal function should refrain from use of these products, even if it has long been considered harmless. Alzheimer's disease would be on the rise where of the aluminum sulphate would have been added to drinking water to make it clearer and more transparent. There are foods that contain aluminum salt including cereals, vegetables, biscuits, dairy products and other foods containing sugar. The aluminum pans increase their toxicity if they are heated to high temperatures. The vaccines contain between 47% to 56% of aluminum. A new-born would receive up to 2.46 mg of aluminum during its vaccines. This phenomenon would have raised the disease of myofascite to macrophage.

The aluminum would cause other health problems including behavior disorders, concentration, irritability, insomnia, anemia, fatigue, colds, colitis, confusion, etc. It affects people differently depending on their rate of health, their weaknesses and their genetic predispositions since it acts as a environmental impact. It attacks the nervous system and also disrupts the assimilation of calcium. The traces of aluminum in dairy products could therefore interfere with the absorption of calcium and thus contribute to the porosity of bone. The aluminum would cause disturbances to the lungs, to the intestines, to the OS, the kidneys, the liver, the stomach and the brain.

"Experiments on rats have shown that the Aluminum accelerates the aging process of the nerve structures of the brain."[274] Since the acid rain are to return to the surface of the ground the aluminum woke up as well any its toxicity and pollutant shallow layers, the fact to consume especially foods that are more acidic than alkaline would render the aluminum even more toxic.

Cadmium

The cadmium would take several tens of years before it can be removed from the body, without forgetting its accumulation over the years. In cervids in Quebec would be contaminated to cadmium, which represents a danger of intoxication for hunters. This toxic metal is deposited on plants that serve as food to these animals, after having been transported in the atmosphere. It is distributed throughout the plant and may not be withdrawn by a simple washing. There are cadmium, among others, in seafood, smelleders, paints, mines, fungicides, the food grown in contaminated soil, tap water and the water of wells, the cigarette smoke. Dolls and other toys of children may contain antimony and cadmium. Cadmium is found everywhere, both in the food that in the air. It is estimated that a human being can consume each day up to 20 micrograms of cadmium.

The danger of this cumulative poison comes from its regular consumption in small quantities. It also would come from agricultural activities since some products used in the fields contain. The cadmium can cause sterility, disorders to the kidneys and the vertebrae, osteoporosis and anemia. It destroys the biology of our cells, damages the nerve cells, because of allergies, neutralizes the amino acids which are at the basis of life and of which their function is the detoxification, product of free radicals, modifies our genetic code, increases as antibiotic bacterial resistance and will supersede the essential minerals. It weakens the immune system and it is also carcinogenic. Genetic damage caused by him would engender congenital malformations. It would cause damage to the nervous system and a curve of growth slowed down.

"With respect to cadmium, it is known that it causes cancer and according to some tests on animals, damage to the kidneys. It may also affect the development of the brain."[275] Regarding the damage to the heart caused by heavy metals, this should ensure that the medical system practice more chelation, which would be more beneficial in the long term that the pumping or coronary other treatments of this kind.

Mercury

The particles of mercury are the most difficult to extract from the body and they can block and prevent the evacuation of other heavy metals and toxins. Mercury is considered toxic since Antiquity.

Human activity diffuse in the atmosphere 70% of emissions of mercury by the exploitation of coal-fired power plants and factories of incineration. This represents nearly 1500 tonnes of emission of mercury per year while knowing that this heavy metal is dangerous for men and animals.[276]

The mercury would be used to treat the skins and furs. Its use in the manufacture of paper, pesticides and medicines is to ensure that its dispersal is felt everywhere in the environment. It would also be in the treated seed, fish, with drugs such as diuretics and purgatives which have resulted in the death of patients, the ointment to treat syphilis, dental amalgam in which it would contain more than what the WHO the would, the bulbs to low energy consumption, the thimerosal in vaccines, antiseptics, thermostats, thermometers, etc. There would be less of mercury in the fish and seafood that in vaccines. It is in would also serve in the laboratories of hospitals. Poultry and eggs may contain mercury if they come from intensive farming and industrial sectors and if they have been fed with Flours of contaminated fish or by food treated with pesticides that contain it. All heavy metals released into the environment by the man can find themselves in the flesh of animals. The animals to drink in the course of water contaminated with mercury. In the fetus, the mercury would concentrate eight times more easily. "Significant quantities of mercury spend of the body of the mother to the fetus. There is also a lot of mercury in breast milk. This poisoning of the young child has for consequences reduced growth, a smaller brain, a immune system and a body weight reduced."[277]

Pollutants such as radioactive particles, dioxins which are carcinogenic, heavy metals, pesticides, insecticides would be in breast milk, but despite everything, it would remain the milk the least polluted.

According to a report of the AFSSAPS (French Agency for sanitary safety of health products), cow milk from which is manufactured the infant formula contains mercury! Therefore, the milk of cow, which is consumed by the whole world (and particularly by the children) contains mercury, and therefore all dairy products.[278] Dairy products may also contain lead and aluminum. The industry of the infant milk formula would be above $8 billion each year, because advertising companies boast about its merits in believing to mothers that it is better to feed her baby with this artificial milk that with its natural milk. Breast milk is a living liquid that best adapts to the needs of the child who develops. It ensures a better brain development. Small concentrations of mercury can have repercussions on the future capabilities (coordination and programming) of the child. The industrial milk would contain more mercury than breast milk. However, the goat milk would prove to be a good replacement product.

Contaminants would remain in the manufacture of infant milk formula. In some commercial preparations for infants, there would have already found the following elements: plasticizers which can be of endocrine disruptors, chemical residue that can come from pesticides and fertilizers, and heavy metals such as lead, cadmium, manganese, the aluminum. In the preparations for infants, there would be significantly greater quantities of manganese, which is a chemical substance neurotoxic, which would have already been put in relationship with attention deficit disorder with or without hyperactivity. The preparations of milk formula soy-based in would contain much more. These formulas would contain six times more cadmium than that of cow, as well as of phytestrogens that act on the thyroid, which can disrupt the endocrine system and weaken the immune system. They could be part of those responsible for the premature development of breasts in girls and reproductive problems in boys.

The majority of the Boxes and packaging used in the distribution of infant formula end up in the waste collection centers that contribute to the pollution of groundwater or are incinerated, which releases toxins carcinogens such as dioxin in the air. The products of feeding infants such as bottles and teats in plastic also end up in the waste collection centers and it is estimated that their degradation will take between 200 to 400 years.[279]

Artificial feeding would cause 260 tonnes of additional waste per year.

The yogurt and cheese would contain 200 times more xénohormones, growth hormones, dioxins, herbicides, pesticides and antibiotics. The milk of cow is made and designed specifically for the needs of the calf and do we should not. The stomach of the human being would not be done to digest milk of cow. We are the only species that continues to drink milk after weaning and more that of another species. It is not a food is also fundamental to the man that makes us believe the agri-food industry. It can therefore cause serious health problems.

The milk cow just as the infant formula would be the cause of ear infections, diarrhea and allergies. The milk other maternal that can produce inappropriate secretions in the infant and decrease the biliary secretion. It cannot be well the digest, absorb or assimilate it without problems. The calcium in milk incorrectly assimilated can become toxic to the body, because it could be transformed into free radicals. The infant milk formula may contain a glutamic acid and aspartic acid that would be recognized as carcinogenic, which could explain the increase in the rate of cancer in children.

The milk is part of acidic foods that contribute to the fixing of toxins, heavy metals and solvents. The heavy metals will fix more easily on a land acid. Dairy products would disrupt the intestinal flora in feeding the yeasts which the love and who also love the land acids. The cheese sticks to the intestines and ferments, which grants a favorable ground for the installation of intestinal parasites pathogens. Rich in saturated fat, milk would be responsible for obesity, gastrointestinal disorders, of ear infections, bronchial disorders, dermatological, rheumatic and joints, genital infections and urinary Same as skin infections such as eczema and respiratory infections, lymphatic disorders circulatory and. Too Rich in proteins, it surstimulerait the parathyroid.

The milk, which is still distributed in primary schools in every morning by some school boards careless, would contribute to the hyperactivity, attention deficit, fatigue leading to the loss of motivation. It would contribute to the loss of language among children and to autism. Since the heavy metals such as mercury destroys the digestive enzymes, leading to an intolerance to lactose or an allergy to the casein, the mercury would be responsible for the increase of peptides in the urine, because it increases the intestinal permeability. Of neurological disorders due to these peptides disrupt the immune system. The milk is part of the three foods most allergens and leads to a self-poisoning by intestinal inflammation that can lead to poor absorption of nutrients and anemia by lack of iron. The casein is a large molecule which would retain in a cluster pasting the nutrients, minerals as well as the toxins and heavy metals. Fruit and vegetables, and Fruits of sea non polluted as well as the nuts are rich in iron. Red meats that stick to the intestines prevent them to absorb the iron they contain. Since the milk and its products are acidifiers, they would lead to a bone demineralization and contribute to the great rate of osteoporosis among the largest consumers of dairy products.

The heavy metals, mainly the mercury(Hg) present in the additives, vaccines, dental amalgam or in the form of vapor as well as the industrial products, can cause damage enzymes in the cycle of cellular respiration or irreversible damage on the nuclear and mitochondrial DNA. It is therefore important not to neglect the action of these heavy metals, responsible for the insurgency of the Hypo and hyperactivity, learning difficulties, dyslexia, of the dysphasia, of the disturbance and the delay of the language, psychomotor delays, behavior disorders ranging up to various autistic symptoms, epilepsy and other diagnostics such as schizophrenia.[280]

The sensitivity to mercury is different from one person to the other. Everyone reacts differently to intoxication to heavy metals: It depends on the genetic predisposition, lifestyle, the unbalanced diet, exposure to other toxins and pollutants, the capacity of detoxification and environmental impacts. The presence of the other heavy metals would render the mercury still more toxic and deadly. It would be in the Agency in combination with other chemical elements. Some bad bacteria would transform the mercury into a substance up to 50 times more toxic. There would therefore be a cause and effect relationship between the viral diseases, fungal and bacterial infections with the deposition of mercury which, acting as an antibiotic very powerful, destroy the intestinal flora whose immune system depends to fight infections, which would allow free course to their development. Thimerosal from vaccines could accentuate the development of Candida.

"There is no of herpes without deposits of mercury."[281]

Although doctors claim that the properties of mercury to the inside of the vaccines are under its form the most innocuous, they have not thought to its transformation into a form more toxic by microorganisms including intestinal yeasts which would transform inorganic mercury into methyl mercury, a more toxic substance, which penetrates more quickly to the tissues of the body of the same as the brain. The mercury would slow down the movement of bile making the bile more thick and sticky. It would therefore be also responsible of the stones in the liver and ulcers in the stomach. The high sensitivity of our nervous system and our organization as a whole to electromagnetic waves depends on the rate of heavy metals in us. They désactiveraient amino acids responsible for detoxification. The dental filling would contain other toxic materials such as money, of tin and copper. The sugar and the fluorine would release more mercury from dental amalgam. It would be the same at each chewing. Remove the gray seal could release more mercury in the system than to keep it. "When the mercury is removed from the body, other toxins escape from themselves. By contrast, as long as the mercury is present, the other toxins must be eliminated one by one."[282]

Among all of the health problems and symptoms caused by the mercury poisoning are found all of the following elements: lesions and damage to the central nervous system, tremor, speech difficulties, excessive salivation with or without burrs, abdominal pain, vomiting, renal failure leading to dialysis more and more young people, damage to the intestines, to the lungs and liver, psychological disturbances, muscle disorders, mood changes, problems to the organs, to other systems and the lymphatic system, degeneration of the spinal cord. In addition, we would: disturbance of the enzyme system, alteration of the structure of the chromosomes, destruction of cellular membranes, allergies, exhaustion of the immune system, neurological damage, disturbance of the digestion, decrease in energy, decrease of the faculties of the reproductive system.

Mercury is a neurobehavioral disruptive, memory, language and concentration. It would be the cause of the mononucleosis, herpes, candidiasis, night sweats, hands and feet cold, autoimmune diseases, multiple sclerosis, tuberculosis, viral infections. It would prevent the viral immunization vaccines, which makes inexplicable its presence in the interior of those. It disrupts the hormones and cognitive functions.

"During autopsies made on persons died of cancer, there was able to find a quantity too high of mercury in the heart of tumors."[283] There is a greater quantity of heavy metals to the inside of the brain tumors. When mercury enters the ducts of our neurons, the power supply to the nerves and the elimination of waste would be compromised, which is that the neurons would become poisoned by their own waste. A land compromises acid detoxification.

Four times more deposition of mercury and two times more deposition of aluminum would have been found in the brains of people who died of Alzheimer's disease. Cancer would have increased in the same time that the use of mercury and aluminum in vaccines.

"Research in Switzerland have demonstrated that by using chelators to eliminate lead from the body, the number of certain forms of cancer could decrease by 90%."[284]

The Mercure expels the essential minerals including zinc and it takes their place within the cells. Even if it was a good power supply, our cells suffer from nutritional deficiencies. This deficiency in vitamins and amino acids aggravates the cognitive capacities. Mercury is toxic, regardless of its concentration, and he cause of psychological disturbance, nerve and muscle. Mercury and lead diminish the capacity of the red blood cells to carry oxygen providing a decrease of energy in the cells. Research scientists have been able to demonstrate that even in small quantities, the mercury can cause damage to the hormones, enzymes, blood cells, the adrenal glands, the pituitary gland, the kidneys, the liver as well as the immune system.

When the mercury from dental amalgam adds to the mercury in vaccines and other products including pesticides, the toxicity increases of as much more if it is in contact with other toxins, heavy metals or agencies that the activate more.

At the University of Calgary, researchers would have proceeded to fillings on teeth of sheep and would have checked the route of mercury with a specialized camera. To the inside of a day, or 24 hours, mercury is would be housed in the spinal cord, brain, kidneys, the hormonal glands, the ovaries, testes, and especially the intestines. It would have accumulated a little everywhere in their body without exit. A dental hygienist has made me believe that mercury evaporated fillings at the time where it is implanted. The order of dentists would have dismissed this study, because it has unfortunately not been made on rats. He must believe that our system would work the same way as that of rodents to the detriment of that of ruminants.

Since the outbreak of autistic symptoms comes, in part, of intoxication to heavy metals, to have the heart net, we have done analyze samples of hair in a laboratory; it was even possible to know the habits of an obese patient in analysing its hair in order to be able to put in place a customized plan. In any case, the analyzes of the hair of our son showed a severe intoxication to arsenic significantly higher than the norm. The arsenic would accumulate, especially in the nails and hair. A high dosage present in samples of hair would indicate a chronic poisoning, because this would give a very good indication of the quantity that can be found in the system. The presence of the tin in his organization also exceeded the average permitted. The aluminum and antimony followed closely the limit of what could be considered as acceptable. Cadmium and lead were arriving respectively in the fifth and sixth position. The rate of mercury was relatively low to our great surprise. The possibilities are the following: The efficacy of homeopathic treatments who cleaned up its system of residues of vaccines, or mercury is remained stuck in its system. Analyzes of blood or stool we would have confirmed. Mercury is the last heavy metal to leave the body and it retains the evacuation of others, therefore its presence in small quantities by the hair analysis indicates a failure of the system of detoxification. In most cases, this are the yeasts, which retain.

By contrast, potassium, manganese, boron, selenium, iron, germanium and rubidium, essential elements in minerals, were at the lowest level in relation to the normal, which will itself since the heavy metals involved are antagonists of essential minerals are missing and that the first dislodged the other to take their place. For example, the high rate of arsenic fact down the rate of selenium. By increasing the selenium by supplements, this allows to combat the arsenic. It must increase the soldiers to fight the other Army. A system in lack of essential nutrients can not well fight against the invaders. It must be that the soldiers are well fed.

The rate of lithium was non-existent. This is a mineral often prescribed in the form of medication to persons suffering from depression or bipolar disorder. This is a mineral that can be found also in the form of supplements, because it is less and less present in our food and his disability is more and more present in children with autism. We rule a good part of the autistic symptoms with supplements appropriate to each case. You can do tests in the laboratory by requesting a keychain levies and by sending a sample of hair for poisoning in the long term, or of blood and stool for poisoning recent.

A chelation in rats has decreased their blood pressure. Heavy metals would cause of cardiovascular diseases. The detoxification to heavy metals is done by a process that is called a chelation. This would be the best antidote. There would be ways to achieve the extraction of heavy metals: Of Injections intravenously under medical supervision that can cause dangerous side effects such as a decrease in the calcium followed by cardiac and respiratory diseases Given that this way Strong does not just take out the heavy metals, but all minerals also essential and at the same time. There is the fresh method which consists of taking natural products harmless as the coriander, Chlorella, garlic, spirulina and flax seed. They act a little like magnets and ensure that the particles of heavy metals to adhere to it, become soluble and are thus evacuated of the body in the urine. The food antioxidants can also help in the evacuation.

To eliminate them in any security, it is not enough to dislodge the heavy metals of these cells, but it must ensure that they will be supported by other biochemical elements who are attracted to them and will lead out of the body in an effective and safe manner.[285]

A chelator composed of Chlorella, an alga specific, can reduce and even eliminate the hyperactivity in a child. Since the beginning of the treatment by natural chelating, our son is no longer never complained of tingling in the eyes. This would confirm the effectiveness of the products, while confirming that it was indeed intoxicated in the tin and mercury. As a result of these treatments by oral chelation, after a few weeks, our son is put to talk more. It became also more lit, more present and more receptive. It has even become Taquin, it is put to love we play of the towers. In addition, it appears to be developed on different aspects and have had a growth spurt, as if, before, something prevented. It is as if he had just to wake up from a nightmare.

In the magazine English-speaking Scientific American and discover to April 2007 in the article "Understanding Autism: The answer may lie in the gut, not in the head" ("understanding autism, the response is located in the intestines, and not in the head"), a child has said to his mother, after having followed a chelation: "Mom, I'm back from death life!" ("Mom, I am income of between the dead!").

Chapter 13

Genetically modified organisms

We are what we eat

Genetically modified organisms (GMOS) could well lead to a form of food poisoning. The genetic changes should, in principle, to improve yields and the resistance to insects and disease while reducing pollution, which is far from always being the case. Scientists wanted to create drought-resistant plants, vegetables which wilt less quickly and can tolerate the climatic and soil conditions poor. Of the animals would have been genetically modified so that they produce more meat and wool. The researchers believed they had found a way to overcome hunger in the world. Slander or speculation? Gmos could well be at the origin of new chronic diseases and incurable. Because of allergies they cause, they could also become responsible for the possible triggering of a new world hunger.

"Say That GMOS are created in order to combat hunger in the world is a pure lie."[286] Therefore, they represent a potential risk to health and the environment. In 2004, 70 per cent of the corn and the genetically modified soybean were cultivated in the world only to feed animals in order that the rich people can have the meat in their base. We are far from overcome the human starvation in the third world. They would use the same of their land, because 8.5 million farmers would use of GMOS which 90% in under-developed countries. Their products would be exported. The peasants would be handled. In addition, nearly 40% of which is cultivated and high ends up in the garbage. Peppers are thrown just because they do not have a beautiful shape.

Before, the improvement of a species met the order of nature that prevented a cow to interbreed with a horse. The genetic manipulation crosses the species barrier by crossing the animal world with the plant world. Scientists play with the basic mechanisms of life.

The genetic modification is a technique where there is a processing non-natural genetic baggage of a living species, that it is of the plant kingdom or animal. It is at the level of the cell, in the center of the latter, that is found the DNA containing the chromosomes.

It is a plant, an animal, a virus, bacterium, unicellular organism or multicellular, or a microorganism which has transformed the hereditary heritage in order to equip it with properties that the nature has not assigned. The genome has been modified in the laboratory by insertion of a gene or genes counterparts (of the same species) or heterologous (from a different species).[287]

This process is done by inserting a gene of synthesis invented by man or that from another species completely different. The transformation is artificial and not natural. It is equivalent to the removal or replacement of one or several genes.

"With respect to genetically modified plants, their DNA has undergone immense violence during the transgenic process, because of the complex manipulations assault their cells."[288] The interaction of genes between them may give rise to unknown functions or the introduction of new genes can wake of genes asleep. In other words, the addition of a gene can change and cause the expression of other genes which would have remained inactive otherwise that can trigger the production of toxins. The insertion of a gene is not always accurate. It can land anywhere, which may reactivate the genes remained silent during millions of years. The transgene in relationship with the other can create a malfunction of the metabolism and create a toxic protein, or inhibit the proteins responsible for the degradation of toxins and cause an accumulation. This forced combination of genes to the interior of a cell is done in a manner so sharp that this can cause interruptions or changes not required in metabolic functions, and this will be very difficult to predict. Therefore, we try and then we shall see what it gives you a time that evil will be done even if this will be irreversible as environmental contamination and food.

We do not know almost never where you place the transgene in the genome receiver not more that one is always absolutely sure not to introduce only one gene. And not only do we do not know where the transgene is fixed, but we do not know when. With the famous cannons in genes, it must release many bursts to shoot at goal.[289]

The genes located around may change its expression. As well, an essential molecule can be accidentally changed. The transgenesis would still not under control as technique. It is difficult to know if the gene has reached its host. The stability and evolution of genes would still be very unrecognized. The result is likely to be unstable. The new gene can disrupt the operation of the plant can result in the production of a new toxin or increase the toxic content of a substance already present, or make a change of place toward the edible part of the plant. New toxic molecules may have been produced as a result of the genetic modification. During this disturbance, the separated molecules could unite to other molecules incompatible that can create a foreign substance and dangerous. We are not immune from a food poisoning. In addition, the insertion of a transgene in the genome of the plant can cause a potential interaction on the functioning of other genes, giving them new functions unknown and unpredictable.

We destroy in so little time that the earth has built during several millions of years. What is done today can create serious health problems in a few decades. The evil will be felt in the long term, as a time bomb. It accumulates in the bodies and creates the dangers latent. This will be our children who in écoperont as well as their descendants. Is that what the next generations could generate mutants monsters?

Gmos could change our own genes, because "we are what we eat"! If these chemicals used in agriculture really alter the DNA of the earthworms, as some studies would show, how could it not be the same concerning our own DNA and the impact of GMOS on this one? If a simple genetic mutation can cause health problems, how can it be beneficial for the beings that feed on? How is it that the food transferred may not cause mutations in the beings who eat? Eat fat makes us big or makes our skin and our hair bold. Or is it that the genetic incompatibility would lead to a new form of infertility? Here are some of the many questions to which I will try to respond a little later.

"The GMOS cause of the types of genetic pollution. These molecules may stick to the DNA, cause mutations in the genetic material and cause cancers."[290] A mutagenic characteristic can become carcinogenic, since the cancer is a change in the functions of the cell to the interior. Even that particles of DNA of bacteria or viruses can unite to other and thus create new diseases by recombination with exchanges of residues. It is worrying to think that medicines would be manufactured from genetically modified bacteria. In principle, a plant virus does not affect the animal world, except by recombination in the crossing of genetic barriers by an artificial process. The GMOS in the production of drugs could involve risks of transmission of pathogens. A generic drug has been genetically modified to make it even more powerful than the original, and there have been several victims of paralysis which have not been able to continue the company, because the patent of invention would have been protected. A human gene of insulin production would have been introduced in an animal to produce human insulin. It would be the same for the production of growth hormones. Of genetically modified bacteria would have been used in vaccines. By inserting a gene in the DNA of a host, its genetic baggage may be damaged, which may lead to pathologies. There are also the risks related to what is called "the horizontal transfer of genes". A cell in contact with another which has been amended can therefore mutate in acquiring the characteristics of the other. The unpredicted side effects may affect now or assign the next generations.

"At the present time, there is no long-term study on the health risks related to the consumption of GMOS."[291] Since GMOS would be badly digested, they would remain in us. They could continue to produce toxins, foreign proteins and pesticides in our intestines and colonize. Of GMOS in the intestines could destroy as well the intestinal flora and enzymes.

A proliferation of cells in the small intestine has been noticed during a study done on rats fed only to genetically modified foods. "The Food transgenic, indigestible, remained frozen in the intestines."[292]

Rats fed only with GMOS have grown up less quickly, but their intestines have become heavier and larger with a weakened immune system. Bacteria and yeasts present in the intestines of bees had absorbed the genetic material of the genetically modified rape, which proves the existence of a horizontal transfer. It would be very surprising that the same thing could not happen to the inside of us.

The power supply of the mother may affect the DNA of her fetus and could lead to pathologies of metabolism once become child or adult such as disorders of the nervous system, immune and digestive systems. Of the jars of food for babies may contain genetically modified food and no one would mention on the label. Certain preparations for infants as infant formulas may also contain. The GMOS can cause allergies and toxic reactions. The genetic modification of a food may make allergen. Combinations of protein molecules can have thus been created artificially to give birth to a new unknown protein which will be rejected by the body. The GMOS may therefore cause allergies and toxic reactions. The introduction too early proteins not natural in the digestive system of a child could cause health problems that could cause an alteration of the digestive functions, enzymatic, nutritional and immune. It must not be forgotten that most of these products have also pushed with fertilizers and pesticides that can represent another form of intoxication, and molecular combination possible, especially if one considers the plants which can produce by themselves now their own insecticides that can destroy our intestinal flora.

If our organization may not recognize the GMOS because they are denatured, it therefore cannot digest properly, nor the absorb, or assimilate their nutrients, and could even trigger of the antibody to the origin of food allergies.

Not to what is not natural

If the wheat, corn, soybeans and rapeseed become the grasses the more genetically modified, one understands why allergies are on the rise as dizzying. The triggering of food allergies could well be a response of the body against the genetic modification. A weakening of the immune system will lead to a gradual poisoning. Strange coincidence with the GMOS, but several autistic children suffer from food allergies many and intolerance of all kinds of even that of intoxication. It would be difficult to ignore the link between autism and GMOS. Guinea pigs which have been fed with peas and beans not genetically modified have not had of allergic reactions. However, the animals fed with peas genetically modified organisms have developed an increase of antibodies in the blood serum and inflammation in the lungs. The introduction of a gene produces a protein new to which we could not adapt.

"In addition, the protein produced by the inserted gene could prove to be toxic or allergenic depending on the capacity of our Organization to the digest or not; release of toxic compounds or allergens for our organization. The use of genes related to known allergens gave them the same characteristics as the latter."[293] This means that the food which receives a gene of a food allergen potentially becomes a food allergen itself. Food allergies are on the increase due to industrialization and the chemical feed and denatured. More and more people are becoming allergic to corn. Of the genetically modified maize has been prohibited for the human food supply and fair for animal consumption, because the protein produced was allergen since it resisted the digestive enzymes. It is very possible that this corn intended for animals has contaminated the fields of corn destined for the human food supply. By contrast, the variation in the amount of protein could trigger allergic reactions. The body may react in a way surprising in the face of a new protein. It would be difficult to predict whether the creation of new proteins will make or not the plant allergen.

"Food allergies are caused by protein which the organization reacts strongly. This are the genes that are responsible for the production of proteins."[294] Therefore, the mixture of new proteins would cause new allergies.

This has become unavoidable when a protein of sunflower seed, that the intention was to substitute to a protein allergenicity of cashew nuts, and who had in addition to the interest of having an amino acid composition more interesting, has been tested on a very large number of people in the United States. Allergic reactions are unexpected were observed while the sunflower seed had never been until then considered allergenic. In addition, the current techniques do not allow to assess the risk of allergies in a reliable manner and objective.[295]

The amino acids are the basis of the life and play with those, it is Play with life. Of the essential amino acids are deleted, and new amino acids may not be metabolized by the system and thus become toxic.

Researchers would have incorporated the gene of a Brazil nuts, regarded as a highly food allergen, to the inside of the soybean to increase its protein content. This could explain the reason for which several people have developed an intolerance to soy. Even if the product would never have been marketed for human consumption, it risk of contaminating neighboring fields by cross-pollination. The animals may become sick. The cows are not accustomed to eat nuts; this are not of the squirrels. It remains no less that they have evidence of the potential dangerousness of GMOS, but despite everything nothing can stop them.

We do not even have the right to know what we eat. Knowing that certain allergies are fatal, this process would therefore play with the lives of the people. If a person develops an allergy to a food because it is genetically modified, it may not be able to consume this new food if it is totally natural and biological or if the production of antibodies The rejects to life? We would begin already to suffer from a food poisoning and a nutrient deficit.

Most of the cereals and fruit and vegetables that are found at the grocery store would be of GMOS and no label does clarify, although a new law might be soon enter into force on this subject. By the genetic modification, some foods have even lost their nutritional values. In addition to cause irritation to the intestines, difficulties of digestion, the production of antibodies and the emergence of allergies, they would also be responsible for a nutrient deficit with all of the health problems that this entails. Some children with autism suffer from a deficit in essential nutrients. The genetic modification of a food would destroy its nutrient values or him would lose a part. The GMOS would therefore be the basis of a malnutrition and deficiencies would require people to eat more, which would explain the increase in the rate of obesity, because the calories as well as the toxins that accompany the processed foods accumulate in fat.

While a was enough fishing in 1950 to absorb a good ration of vitamin A, it should be today in a chewable twenties. Where are the past these vitamins? The modern orange contains five times less iron. The intensive use of pesticides, herbicides and fertilizer increases the speed of growth of plants and decreases proportionally the time of fixing of micronutrients. Agricultural techniques that intensive deplete the soil; conservation treatments and time of transport; picking of fruits before ripening, in part or totally devoid of nutrients related to the sunshine as anthocyanins or polyphenols, these components who protect us against the cancer or the deterioration of the cells of the brain; practice of selection of plants according to their performance: the higher the return, less the plant expenditure of energy to absorb trace elements, and the more the nutrient content is low.[296]

The death of food

The organic foods that are not genetically modified are more tasty and nutritious. In arriving at maturity too quickly, the foods have less of taste and they have a loss in the nutrient values. A change to improve Vitamin A can cause a deficit in another vitamin D all the more important, or among a protein as well as deficiencies in minerals. How to stop the famine in the world with less nutritious food? In 2001, 20 million adults and 13 million children lived in a food insecurity. In the United States, 10.7 per cent of households are victims of malnutrition.

In response to the insertion of the foreign gene, the plant could generate additional substances that could harm our assimilation of nutrients (vitamins, iron, etc.) present in the plant. Similarly, the insertion of the foreign gene could be a decrease in the content of nutritional substances themselves.[297]

The fact that our digestive system may not recognize a modified DNA makes the food indigestible whose few nutrients which remains can not be assimilated. The foreign gene from a bacterium could unite to other bacteria in our intestine and continue to produce of the insecticide in us which kills the good bacteria in our intestinal flora. "The Soya RR patent contains 27% more of an inhibitor of a digestive enzyme of the pancreatic juice which has for purpose to digest proteins. This may therefore inhibit the digestion of certain proteins and can retard the growth of animals."[298]

During the storage, of food can produce aflatoxins which can also cause health problems for humans as of cancers, liver problems and a hormonal disturbance. There would also be the risk of poisoning by consumption of meat from animals which have been fed with GMOS because of the quantity in insecticides in their flesh which can come modify or destroy our intestinal flora. A gene for resistance to antibiotics ingested in a host cell can be transmitted to the intestinal flora in the body which consumes. We poison to small fire by ingestion of pesticides, herbicides and insecticides. There is therefore an accumulation of these products through the food chain. Of vital organs modified and of the immune defenses weakened were found in rats fed with genetically modified potatoes.

Sheep and goats would be dead after grazed in a field where was cultivated cotton genetically modified. A food genetically modified can therefore be transformed into a kind of poison.

Yet, two thirds of the transgenic plants are genetically modified to produce or tolerate of pesticides, and therefore toxic products for some agencies, whose residues, particularly fat soluble, are likely to accumulate in the food chain and to have toxic effects in the long term.[299]

Some parts of several plants are not edible and are even poisons: the leaves of rhubarb and potato sprouts. Therefore, a genetic modification could deflect this poison to the edible part of the plant; this would then be a true catastrophe world scientific. Even the tomato plants would produce a toxin. The consumption of transgenic foods can lead to a resistance of antibiotics as well as to the allergies with the risk of toxicity which is attached.

"However, a genetically modified food could contain a greater amount of toxins or allergens as a result of the possible reactions of the plant to the insertion of a gene introduced into its genome, including the production of the protein, or proteins."[300] Genetically modified plants contain inhibitors of digestive enzymes, which can make the new toxic proteins. With all the problems arising from the gluten, it would be very difficult to believe that the wheat is not genetically modified. The allergic reaction to soy amended with genes of the Brazil nuts was even stronger with this soybean that with the Brazil nuts only. The GMOS may therefore be more toxic than the originals.

We are far from being in the shelter of the scientific errors that accumulate

The Bt toxin which would come from pesticides used on GMOS has been found in the blood of pregnant women, which represents a danger to the fetus and the unborn baby. Its presence has also been levied in umbilical cords. "The Bt toxin is introduced into the body not only through the direct consumption of GMOS, but also by eating meat, milk, eggs from animals which the power supply contains GMOS."

More than 90 per cent of the children can be contaminated by the toxin Bt. Thirty million hectares of genetically modified plants are grown on the planet. Cross-pollination between genetically modified plants and natural plants contaminate neighboring fields producing fruit and vegetables to biological agriculture that it would be difficult to maintain as well. It is as if there was nothing more to completely organic. The nature will always be stronger than we.

Some agricultural producers qualify their culture of biological. They say that the genetic modification is a natural process since crosses occur in nature without intervention of man. Although the beings of the same species can mate, it is impossible that the nature mates a body of the animal kingdom with a the plant reign without cause of disaster. The salmon would have been genetically modified so that it becomes more large and that it is resistant to colder waters.

A person who is allergic to fish could die by eating a tomato, which has been amended with the gene of a fish. That is why labelling GMOS should be mandatory.

For example, to make the strawberries more resistant to frost, we can collect a fish gene arctic, therefore accustomed to live in icy waters, and introduce in the genetics of strawberries. They then develop with this peculiarity, frost resistance, that they did not have before the Registry of the gene.[301]

It is difficult to believe that we do not serve as guinea pigs. We are even more certain of what we eat, and yet we have the right to know. All genetically modified foods should bear the word GMOS on their label with descriptions of what the food is crossover.

Researchers would have inserted a gene from a bacterium living in the soil to the inside of the genetic makeup of the corn. They had discovered that this bacterium could release a substance that kills the insects. They wanted as well as the maize may emanate itself this insecticide. Yet, this bacterium is not part of our food habit. Person, or almost, has thought about the serious consequences on the health and on the environment. They would have also invented a species of corn that would stand up to the herbicide the more powerful to be able to use in greater quantity and thus pollute more.

The gene of a salmon from the Pacific would have been inserted in the egg of a Atlantic salmon to activate a growth hormone in order it to grow more quickly and that it can resist the cold. This can have a dramatic impact on the terrestrial biodiversity and aquatic. Use of enclosures located in full sea can cause accidents. The genetically modified fish are either infertile or their offspring does not to adulthood; therefore there would have an impact on the hormones.

During a cloning, it transfers the full kernel of a cell to the interior of another cell from the same be in the goal to imitate the fertilization and for that to be in question retains its own genetic background. A nuclear technique would be used in this sense. We have only to remember the disastrous experience conducted once on of the sheep. The cloned animals suffer much. Did you know that the sale of the meat from cloned animals intended for human consumption would have been permitted in the United States recently?

If the allergies to dairy products are today many, then we must ask if this is not because of this with what the cows are fed. Before, they ate of the grass in the fields and drank the water. Today, they remain locked on the inside and are fed with fish meal, cereals GM full of pesticides, and they would receive of growth hormones and antibiotics. That is what the man has done with the milk which would have made if bad. "An increase in the content of uric acid of the meat or milk would be very worrying, because the uric acid is a powerful stimulant for the production of cholesterol in humans."[302]

Would we be ready to eat plants or of the meat which contain human genes? Could it be that one day we in Vienna to transfer a part human genetics in the plants? If the government uses the money of taxpayers to fund experimental research, then we are working without the knowledge, with our taxs, and to our own destruction. Why not fund rather research to address the causes of autism instead of contributing to its expansion? It is ripped off. We are tanned to hear that there is no scientific study of made to this subject when there are several, but we prefer to do a deaf ear.

Genetic pollution

The risks have not been assessed and the GMOS already cause enormous evils. The genetically modified plants can mix their genes with wild herbs of the same family and make those resistant to the herbicide. "A genetically modified plant can perfectly transmit the new genes to another neighboring plant transgenic non-belonging to the same species, what is called genetic pollution."[303]

This transmission from plant to plant is not controllable. By crossing spontaneous, cultivated plants can exchange their genes with a related wild species, which risk of creating weeds, thus creating a genetic pollution which will be irreversible. The contamination of neighboring fields is already uncontrollable and difficult to control. Rapeseed without GMOS would not exist almost more in this country because of the genetic pollution. The erucic acid is 10 times greater in the rapeseed today that in the former species. A plant which emanates continuously from the insecticide pollutes more than the methods of before which consisted in spreading occasionally. This pollution eventually ends up in our plates and in the air. There is an accumulation of more and more of herbicides and insecticides in the food chain. Genetic pollution can lead to a food poisoning.

The scientists are still ignorant of the impact of the genetic modification on the nature, on the environment including the flora and fauna, and on the health of all living beings. The profitability and the quantities take precedence over the quality and health.

In the transgenic soybean the Monsanto corporation, a gene introduced makes the plant tolerant to a herbicide total (because it kills all plants, good or bad), the Roundup marketed by the same company. In a natural culture, the use of herbicides is limited because the cultivated plant in also suffers. The soybeans being rendered tolerant to the herbicide Roundup, it is possible to considerably increase the doses, causing increased pollution of soils and groundwater.[304]

This could introduce new generations of insects, parasites and weeds ultra-resistant. Pesticides should be used in larger quantities. The contamination of the food chain will be even more important since the insecticide or herbicide is located on the inside of the plant and not only to the outside such that with the old methods of spreading. Therefore, wash the food or remove its skin does not protect us.

It should be noted that the farmers using soybeans of Monsanto have the obligation not to use that his herbicide, the Roundup. As well, Monsanto sells its transgenic seed and strongly increases its sales of herbicides, reflecting the concern for the profitability of agrochemical firms to the detriment of the environment.[305]

This herbicide would not be biodegradable and would accumulate in the soil and water courses as well as groundwater by percolation. Farmers suffer from neurological disorders such as Parkinson's and Alzheimer's diseases or paralysis. Of the Indian peasants ruined commit suicide. The farmers do not have the right to use the grains of plants for planting the following year and are forced to buy, which impoverishes, because otherwise their products would be blocked by the food industry. It is a big lobbying.

The GMOS had to decrease the agricultural pollution, while it is the reverse effect.

Government studies show an increase of 15 times the use of herbicide Roundup (glyphosate) in the United States and almost 80 per cent in Brazil. This is linked to the increasing number of weeds resistant to glyphosate everywhere in the world, thus increasing the costs of production and the environmental impacts. The United States have also increased their use of pesticides more toxic, one of which is banned in Europe.[306]

The cultivated land with GMOS have increased by 75% since 1996. Would it be possible to feed 10 billion people in 2050 without environmental degradation irreversible? This represents a threat to world food security. Approximately 80% of the corn planted in North America is GMOS. The toxin of transgenic maize BT would contaminate the sediments at the bottom of the St. Lawrence River and in the other courses of water. "Scientists have observed that the sediments from the St. Lawrence (at the mouth of the Richelieu) contained concentrations five times higher of the Bt toxin that the drainage waters."[307]

The GMOS may create the vagaries of food. Fruit and vegetables as well created have less of taste. They lose their original flavor which gave us both the taste to eat. When animals have the choice to eat a GM food or natural, they avoid by instinct the bowl which contains GMOS and are more attracted to the natural food. They would be willing to eat not to die of hunger if they are the only food that is given to them. Experiments conducted on laboratory rats have shown that the animals are more attracted to healthy foods by those who have been modified. Our children may not have lost this instinct of survival.

The meat could contain more pesticides that fruit and vegetables by bioaccumulation throughout the chain. The conditions of intensive livestock production to ensure that the flesh of animals concentrated more pesticides and more quickly because of their fattening and of their rapid growth which are such that they do not have the time to detoxify their system. Their organization has a lower capacity to eliminate the pesticides because of their inappropriate power supply. This whole food pollution is not just accidental, but it is voluntary by ignorance and disbelief. Processed foods contain too many chemicals.

By the genetic modification, plants have lost their natural means of defense. The genetic transformation of a product would make them more vulnerable to new parasitic infections, viral or bacterial.

When the natural corn is attacked, it emanates a substance that attracts of insect predators and parasitic diseases to help him. It is a natural defense that it loses with the genetic modification.

All insect pollinators could therefore be victims of poisoning to pollen insecticide. The pollen would be polluted and contaminated by the transgenic DNA which could change the genetic makeup of bees in acting on their behavior. Of the substances may change the behavior of living beings. Traces of transgenic DNA have been found in hives deserted.

The bees and other insects are endangered. A large percentage of hives are deserted. The pesticides in their would lose the sense of direction or the intoxiqueraient simply, such an ant who reports a fourmicide in its nest which kills all the ants which the Queen. Another possibility would be that the bees not recognizing the plants transformed by the hand of man, refuse to touch it and lack of pollen to their larvae who die. The pollen is also transported by the wind and the water droplets, which risk of contamination to other plants and other fields.

What are the doses of insecticides and herbicides which are found as well in our plates? A summer, every time that my husband and I ate corn cobs expense, the next day, we were in a very bad mood. Therefore, pesticides can have an impact not just on the behavior but on the mood. What can we say of the increase of violence in the school and the crime rate in society?

A real disaster

By killing the earthworms, responsible for the aeration of the soil, the latter risk to compress further. The chemicals used on agricultural land would take 10 to 30 years before to be completely broken down by soil organisms that these products destroy. If one considers the accumulation that occurs over the years as well as the quantity of microorganisms killed, the rate of toxic products in the soil would exceed long since the recommended standards.

Animals which have been fed only with genetically modified foods would have suffered from multiple disorders including cancer, as well as lesions of the organs. The SOYBEANS Roundup would a dysregulation in the cells of the liver, pancreas and testes; an increase in white blood cells to the detriment of the red blood cells, an increase of fats and sugar in the blood as well as an inflammation of the liver, kidney problems with lesions in the pancreas and a disruption of the functions of the liver. The kidneys, the liver and intestines are the first to react to the result of a food poisoning chemical. The pigs would have become sterile after

185

having eaten genetically modified maize. Farmers have been hospitalized after having been in contact with pesticides.

The International Council for Science indicates, in 2003, that the GMOS commercialized are more dangerous for human health. By contrast, a study of 2011 indicates that the consumption of cereals or of protein crops genetically modified organisms could cause problems in the kidneys and liver in mammals.[308]

The GMOS may also cause a drop of digestive enzymes. If the GMOS are toxic to animals, they must also be for us. If the GMOS interfere with the target organs for the detoxification of the body of animals, their flesh must then contain enough of toxins to make sick the beings who feed on it. They would also have effects on the heart, the adrenal glands, blood cells and the spleen. Of the animals would be genetically transformed for that their organs are transplanted into humans.

Genes for resistance to insecticides act by disrupting the digestive system of the parasite and act as inhibitors of enzymes. The same thing can then occur in mammals, including humans, that eat the plants containing this insecticide: they have a disturbance of the enzyme system and the problems of digestion. The genetically modified soybean could alter the cells. The consumption of soybeans resistant to the herbicide would make a modification of the kernel of the cells of the liver.

"Then it gives to these mice of soybean non-genetically modified during a month. This change in diet causes a return to the typical characteristics of the nucleus of cells."[309] The surface of the nucleus of cells of the liver is lower among the mice fed the genetically modified soybean that the mice fed with soybeans not genetically modified. Therefore, if the food regimes can affect the structures of the components of the cells, it can affect the functioning of the organs and systems. What we eat can change our DNA and cause all kinds of anomalies such as those caused by GMOS.

Of infertilités would have occurred among mouse embryos fed with GMOS: even sterility that GM plants themselves, which is very disturbing for the reproduction of human beings as well. The researchers have also discovered in these mice accelerated aging, alterations to the principal organs as well as the gastrointestinal system and disorders related to insulin. Almost all reject fed with the GM soybeans die after three weeks. They come in the world more small, in more small number and do not arrive to reproduce. The GMOS may therefore be responsible for the decline in the birth rate of the human being and the increase in the rate of infertility, as well as the deterioration of health in general in humans.

All sheep fed with plants of Bt cotton are dead in the 30 days, and those who pâturaient on plantations of natural cotton have remained in good health. The autopsies revealed a great irritation and black spots at the time in the intestines and in the liver (as well as the bile duct enlarged).[310]

In the same conditions, buffalo died three days after. A million people would be poisoned each year and 22 000 people can die because of this culture. Cotton crops represent 25% of the global use in pesticides. Approximately 65 000 tonnes of pesticides would be sprayed only in France each year on this plantation. The pesticides used on cotton would be part of the most dangerous substances.

"The corn Bt has also been involved in the death of cows in Germany, and horses, buffaloes and chickens in the Philippines."[311]

In humans, there is a strong increase of gastro-intestinal disorders since the last 10 years, as well as chronic diseases. Measurable changes have been discovered in the blood of people with autism. The GMOS are therefore likely to cause problems nutrients, of new diseases, the transfer of genes from one bacterium to another, poisoning and, of course, allergies as well as a change in our genetic background.

"The NK 603 maize, for example, leads to an increase in the weight of the heart and kidney leaks. Regarding the MY 810, in addition to the effects on the liver and kidneys, it causes an average increase of 18 per cent of the weight of the spleen." An increase in blood glucose levels would have been noticed in rats fed with genetically modified Corn Monsanto, as well as an increase in lymphocytes and a high activity in the synthesis of proteins in mice fed exclusively of transgenic soybean. The genetically modified plants also represent a danger for the courses of water.

Traces of the Bt toxin were collected in 23% of the rivers tested. These residues can generate genetic effects secondary which are unexpected. They may contaminate the genetic heritage of terrestrial and aquatic.

A war of good sense

By the artificial modification of the genetic heritage, there will soon have no more healthy food on Earth. We risk losing a large plant diversity, as well as the origin of some living beings. Cross an animal species with a plant species risk of compromising the food chain, which would lead to the disappearance of several hundreds of animal species. The genetic modification would be even stronger than the nuclear and would already have been used as a chemical weapon.

How to protect human fertility when the genetically modified maize affects reproduction in mice with a declining birth rate and the body weight at birth? Is this not already the case among us?

The offspring of rats fed genetically modified soya shows a mortality multiplied by five, a birth weight below and the inability to reproduce. The new sperm cells of male mice fed genetically modified soya are damaged. Among the progeny of mice fed with GMOS of soybeans, the DNA of the embryo has a altered physiology. Several U.S. farmers have reported the sterility or problems of fertility in cows and pigs fed with varieties of genetically modified maize. In addition, in the course of the last two months, investigators in India have informed of fertility problems, abortions, of premature births and other serious violations of the health, including of the dead among the buffaloes fed products to cotton seeds genetically modified.[312]

The plants more genetically modified soybeans, corn, cotton and canola. If the GMOS and pesticides are responsible of the rate of infertility in the populations of the plant kingdom and animal, they can therefore be responsible also other genetic disorders, even that of cancers. The GMOS affect the messages of the cells that can disrupt the rate of hormones, which cause changes in the sexual behavior. Lectins absorbed by the blood can cause metabolic changes resulting in abnormal immune responses and hormonal alterations.

The genetically modified soybean may alter the liver cells and those of the testicles to changes in the color of the latter. These products pollute the soil and can make disappear insects as well as native plant species. There is a tremendous danger of extinction of natural species in the flora and fauna in the wild. Even the farmed salmon genetically modified grows and grows more quickly, but it saw less long.

The Red List of species in danger of extinction published by the IUCN provides us with figures staggering. In 2004, a bird on eight, a mammal on four, an amphibian on three, three insects on four and eight crustaceans are threatened with disappearance [...]. Scientists believe as well very seriously that 15 to 50 per cent of animal and plant species could have disappeared from the face of the Earth by fifty years [...] the disappearance of a species, even modest and of little apparent importance, can condemn all those who depend on it, predators who will no longer have nothing to eat, parasites which disappear with their host, plants that depend on it for their spread. This phenomenon is called co-extinctions. The disappearance of some species can therefore ruining the functioning of the ecosystem inducing a snowball effect uncontrollable.[313]

More than 15 000 species would be endangered and up to 100 000 species to disappear all years. Among the reasons for the disappearance of the species would be the competition of species better adapted to the changes in climate and environmental conditions, hunting, predators, disease resistance, without forgetting the poor adaptation to human actions reckless.

The depletion of biodiversity creates natural plants less resistant to chemicals. Implement a species outside of its natural ecosystem led to an ecological catastrophe and causes the disappearance of other plant and animal species, because it is all their ecosystem which is upset. An ecological imbalance can cause the invasion of a plant or an animal harmful. Therefore, all living beings may be disrupted.

Before, it was the inversion of the Earth's magnetic fields, the drift of the continents, the salinity of the oceans, the modification of the atmosphere and the rate of oxygen in the air and the water, the fall of meteorites, climate change, volcanic eruptions and the lack of food that have changed the conditions of the environment and several species have not been able to adapt quickly enough. The survivors who have been able to adapt have created new species. Despite the progress of medicine, the life expectancy of humans would have declined since 1975.

The causes of extinctions today are: the mass destruction of forests, urbanization, intensive agriculture, pollution, hunting, climate change, as well as the disruption of natural ecosystems that survived before their balance is weakened.

Some environmentalists believe that GMOS would become responsible for the resistance to antibiotics. Gmos are used in the manufacture of pharmaceutical products and medicines. We do not know several long-term effects of drugs as well as their interaction after a certain amount of different kinds. What are the issues to the result of the use of GMOS in the manufacturing of vaccines?

"In Europe, there has been of the scientists who have implanted a dog gene in the genome of corn, which can produce the gastric lipase, a drug. In an open environment, GMOS can disperse by machinery, transportation, birds, bees, wind, etc."[314]

A gene resistant to an antibiotic would have been introduced in corn. The antibiotic resistance genes would have often been used as markers to check if the genetic manipulation has been successful. They would use of antibiotics also to kill all bacteria that have not received the transfer, as well as the residues of the DNA of bacteria. The transfer of genetic material of viruses and bacteria to other plants, even from the dead cells, could make to the long of vaccines inactive.

"Many scientists fear that the dissemination of antibiotic resistance genes from the genetic plants and manipulated only accelerates the process leading to the appearance of pathogenic bacteria against which antibiotics would be powerless."[315]

Residues of genes that have not been used may be transferred to other agencies. The use of a gene for resistance to antibiotics, by consumption, may, in the digestive system of animals and humans, transfer this resistance gene to bacteria making the Antibiotics ineffective. There would therefore be of antibiotic resistance genes in our intestines. Genes for resistance to antibiotics can be found in the food chain. The resistance to antibiotics kills thousands of people each year. The resistance to antibiotics can be transmitted of plants to pathogenic bacteria and cause health problems.

On the subject of other forms of resistance, the rats are not good pets to assess the toxicology of a product because they have become, in the course of generations, immunized and resistant to the rat poison. And rodents does not age at the same speed that we, which fact that their metabolism does not work in the same way at a certain time.

Doctors advise us to avoid GMOS. "The genetically modified soya is so dangerous that I say to the people of never eat."[316]

Without studies nor valid tests measuring all the impacts in the short, medium and long terms, children and adults are used as guinea pigs. The GMOS represent risks for the health since it is fact that begin to discover their side effects. They have been marketed without knowing the impacts. 40% to 60% sprayed products do not reach the plants or soil and remain in suspension in the air. This is not for nothing that the farmers to protect themselves in the enclosing in tractors with cab closed. And we, where are our protective bubbles?

Chapter 14

The hormones

The genetic engineering: another scientific error

It should ask if the hormones that are found in the food can be harmful to our children and their descendants. A hormone would consist of a protein composed of amino acids, and we have seen in the previous chapter that it is dangerous to play with the protein and amino acids.

Of livestock for slaughter or to the dairy production would receive of growth hormones which would come from a genetic modification with a soil bacterium. "A fragment of the human DNA containing the gene encoding the human growth hormone has been isolated, purified, and introduced into the genome of the bacterium Escherichia coli. The bacteria use the human gene and produce of the human growth hormone."[317]

This genetic manipulation of the gene responsible for the production of hormones has been introduced into a bacterium by researchers working for Monsanto, this bad Engineering who would have had to remain locked in its bottle.

Let the dead rest in peace

Other hormones for growth would have already been collected in the past directly in the pituitary gland of some corpses, which were of people who died of... we did not know what. The pituitary gland is a main gland of the nervous system. Mortuary would have been devastated so that we can obtain the pituitary glands; it was another idea of Pasteur, the inventor of the vaccines. There would have been 1200 removed glands around 1984 in morgues of France.

The cause of death of the donor was of little importance. Pickers were paid to the unit. One hundred and ten-Seven deaths have been recorded in children who have received this growth hormone manufactured from levy on the corpses until 1988. "A first serious problem occurred with the production of growth hormones by extraction of corpse, which has caused a number of contamination by pathogens Prions and caused the fatal cases of the Creutzfeldt-Jakob Disease."[318]

This disease can take up to 30 years to develop, which fact that the rate of real victims increases.

The bodybuilding in animals

Growth hormones would be injected or incorporated in the food for the animals in order to increase their body mass to the inside of a much shorter period. Hormones data would be to cows in order that they produce more milk. Growth hormones beef would be used outside of Europe to stimulate production of the dairy cows. They would be used for the meat of animals in order to reduce the

191

cost of production. Today, in 38 days, a chicken is ready to be eaten, whereas before it took three months. The big dairy production would reduce the price of milk, but this would be at the price of our health. The third of dairy cows in the United States receive and their milk would be exported to Canada. The quantity of milk premium on quality. When the American cow is increased from 12 pounds of milk per day to 50 books, it is difficult to believe that this milk contains as much of concentrate nutritious. The BEEF grows 10 times faster. In humans, the growth hormone would have been used for the purpose to keep an eternal youth.

Not guilty, these poor animals

The cow is made to give milk a few months after see calved, and not during the entire year, which runs counter to the nature. Force the cow to produce more milk than its natural capacity can put his life in danger. This disrupts the natural cycle of the cow. Normally, it increases its production of milk to feed her calf, which decreases naturally when the calf grows and that it begins to eat the grass. Before, the cows ate grass peacefully in the fields in the sun; today, they are imprisoned for life attached to chains or Carcans in barns where they cannot even run. This greatly affects the well-being of the animal. It will soon be their prescribe antidepressants and tranquilizers, whose traces of drugs such as all other chemical products that they receive will be in the milk we boirons, hoping that the traces of antidepressants that could contain the milk at that time will not push the people nor the cows to commit suicide.

In a traditional dairy farm, it must therefore be inseminated The Cow of again to restart the cycle of milk production. But the injection of Prosilac allows you to artificially maintain the manufacture of milk beyond the natural cycle of the cow. One of the consequences of breaking the cycle is a decrease in the fertility rate of the animal sometimes ranging up to sterility.[319]

And what is the human infertility among the major consumers of dairy products? The Prosilac would act as a strong drug to the same title that crack whose judgment would cause a shock if large in cows which die by inability to undergo the withdrawal. Would this be one of the reasons for which the children, heavy drinkers of milk, have as much difficulty to concentrate at school and to check? Is that what it would also explain the rate of drug addiction in society? In any case, one understands why people love both the dairy products.

"Milk production increases by an average of 11% to 16%, the clinical risk of mastitis increases of approximately 25%, the fertility decreases of 40% and the clinical risks to develop a limp increase of 55%"[320] These cows on the Prosilac would have put to the world of monstrous calves with the stomach out or with the tabs on the head. Growth hormones would not create any fair of malformations in the fetus of cows, but they cause also among they an increase of cystitis to the ovaries, problems to the uterus, a decrease in the gestation of calves, fever, digestive disorders, indigestion, diarrhea, lesions in the PIS with tissue necrosis.

There is nothing completely white

This excessive production would create of bleeding which may be found in the milk requesting the use of another chemical process in order to separate the blood of the milk for better the extract. In addition, cows are likely to suffer more of mastitis that can leave traces of pus in the milk, which would also increase the taking of antibiotics.

In addition, these problems of mastitis have a different impact on the quality of the milk to treat such inflammations, farmers have recourse to injections of antibiotics whose residues are found in the milk. These same antibiotics then find themselves in the body of the consumer and participate in the development of the pathogenic strains resistant to antibiotics.[321]

These hormones can cause many diseases to cows forcing the use of antibiotics first by way of prevention and then in a manner curative. Approximately 52 kinds of antibiotics have been found in milk in the United States.

The antibiotic residues in milk have increased. Not surprising that children are as much of ear infections. The risk concerning the abuse of the use of antibiotics also acts on the growth of the man. Although the growth hormones are not permitted in some countries, the antibiotics are used, them, as growth promoters.

"The producers gave 20 times more antibiotics that 30 years ago. In all, in the farms of animals, it uses 100 times more of antibiotics that in human medicine."[322] The antibiotics would be used in pig production and for the poultry to increase the growth of animals by stimulating their appetite. The antibiotics in milk kill the good lactic acid bacteria to the detriment of the poor; this would be one of the reasons for which they must add of Lactobacillus in yogurt. The bad bacteria in the intestines of consumers.

In pig farming, 10% are used for the treatment, 53% for the prevention and 43% as a growth promotant [...]. Health Canada is aware that the use of four antimicrobials as growth promoters in

farm animals destined for the human food supply has been banned in the European Union. They are moreover still allowed here.[323]
The antibiotic resistance in humans
Therefore, the antibiotics given to animals would be mainly used as growth promotants. In 2009, more than 1000 tonnes of antibiotics have been administered to livestock.

These antibiotics create a antibiotic resistance. These pacemakers of antibacterial growth have been refused in Europe because their structure is too similar to antibiotics used in human medicine, and growth hormones have been banned in Europe for the livestock because of the risk of cancer that they represent. The antibiotics given to animals can make resistant Salmonella and it can transfer this resistance to other bacteria.

"The United States, for example, evaluate to more than 100 000 the number of U.S. patients who die each year as a result of bacterial infections resistant to all known antibiotics."[324] No study has been able to demonstrate that there is no risk in the long term on the animals, the environment and human health as a result of the use of these products. Of Quebecers would have boasted of having imported a kind prohibited here and who can do fatten more calves more quickly. Despite the prohibitions, there is a parallel market and clandestine, even that veterinarians conscientious little would the traffic of antibiotics and would prescribe without even having seen the animal.

They administer antibiotics to prolong the life of a animal very productive. All of these antibiotics would find themselves in the milk and meat that we eat. This is the reason for which the milk may be responsible for repetitive infections because of the antibiotic resistance and the destruction of the intestinal flora.
Obesity
Children today are much larger than their grandparents. It is in North America that would be the highest rate of obesity, especially among children. When growth hormones are taken continually through the power supply or otherwise, they can produce an effect of gigantism. The overweight of these risk of the drive toward juvenile diabetes and can lead to cardiovascular complications. Growth hormones can grow the heart. Acromegaly is a disease which causes the magnification of the organs and different parts of the body including the Nose And the bones of the face. "Obesity can be linked to hormonal disorder."[325]
Miracle or mirage?

The hormones act on the thyroid gland in affecting its own production of hormones. The autism and ADHD may result from a disorder of the thyroid gland. In the world, 200 million people suffer from disorders of the thyroid. It plays a role in the digestive tract and on the brain being responsible also delays intellectuals. The synthetic hormones can inhibit the uptake of iodine necessary to the functions of the thyroid gland.

The hormones could do swell our organs and inflate the joints as well as cause of the blisters in the face. If a child does not need to produce growth hormones because he receives in his power, his hormones will become ineffective in the Cellular reproduction. They create enlargements to cells, thus creating confusion in the cells. They are acting directly on the tissues of cells. The hormones are a threat to the people most likely to be affected such as pregnant women and children close to puberty. The girls become more pubescent young people.

The thymus, a gland playing a crucial role in the functions of the immune system, may be reduced as a result of the taking of growth hormones, even by the power supply. An immune system damaged prevents people to defend themselves against infections or cancer .

The role of the hormones of growth would also imply the control of proteins. A string of different amino acids produced as well may alter proteins and interact with the functions of the immune system. Rats have developed antibodies against the bovine somatotropin, this growth hormone, during experiments. "Unfortunately, the major part of the American milk contains the viruses of leukemia, tuberculosis, the virus bovine immunodeficiency."[326]

Growth hormones would not cause just of intestinal disorders among the cow whose diarrhea, but also among the one who drink. The milk sugar imbalance also our intestinal flora. "The milk is the cause of allergies, colic, colitis, ear infections, colds and congestion in young children."[327]

Growth hormones affect all metabolism, result in the loss of amino acids, affect the synthesis of proteins, create an increase in fat, a mobilization of lipid reserves, and also exercise a peptide function which acts on the receivers. They can cause tendinitis, diabetes and pre-diabetes, influence the breathing capacities and increase the rate of cholesterol.

The peptide of bovine albumin can cause diabetes in humans. In addition, it would be responsible of anomalies to the peripheral nerves and those located at the ends, an increase in the rate arterial, pain in the legs and muscles as well as erectile dysfunction in the consumers of steroids. The albumin would be used in the manufacture of vaccines. An excess of growth hormones can cause osteoarthritis. The milk can cause the juvenile acne by overproduction of fat Fat in the blood and increase the dental caries by his acid pH; it promotes of allergies and the problems of growth among children. The danger comes from the ingestion of these substances to repetition.

The hormones of growth would have been given to patients in hospitals in the hope that they heal more quickly, but it would not have made that increase the rate of mortality and the period of hospitalization.

A unbalanced balance

The estrogen content in the milk of cows would create hormonal imbalances. Hormones play a role in sexual and social behavior as well as on the mood, anxiety, hyperactivity, sleep disorders and the aggressiveness. The interaction between the hormones and the thyroid functions would play a role in the Depression. The hormones would be of endocrine disrupters because a too high rate of a certain kind of hormones would influence the production of the other. Andropause and menopause generate mood swings inexplicable and of antisocial and aggressive behavior, stronger in some people. The hormones cause a feminization of males and a decline in libido among women. Everything to promote the reproduction. The sexual behavior even in animals is changed because the too high rate of synthetic hormones that are found in the rivers female condition here the fish.

If this are mostly boys who are with autism, is there not here a direct link with the hormones that are found in the power supply, especially if the presence of these hormones can affect the metabolism to the point of preventing the extraction of heavy metals outside of their system? Then, again, the supply would be a source of intoxication.

The regulation of our hormones of production may be disrupted by the presence of growth hormones and generate infertilités such as for the COW, since we drink the milk and we eat its meat which may contain traces. More and more calves die at birth. The cows that are no longer productive enough end at the slaughterhouse. The toxic effects of growth hormones in beef, some of which are imported, would play a role on human fertility. These residues of hormones in the flesh of animals can break the endocrine balance.

The hormones play a role in cancer of the pancreas, thyroid and Intestines including that of the colon. They would also create tumors in the pituitary gland. "Hormones used in beef production in Canada such that oestradiol, progesterone, testosterone, the trembolone, zeranol Melengestrol Acetate (MGA) are in effect to all suspected to stimulate the growth of tumors."[328]

They could be responsible of tumors of the genital organs, of the liver and pancreas, and cause testicular abnormalities. Growth hormones would act on the cells of the liver. We could cure well of breast cancers by stopping to consume dairy products. That stimulates the production of milk in the cow can cause the same effect on the cells of the breast of women. "A study published in the Harvard's Physicians Health Studies and conducted on 12 000 men indicates an increase of 43 per cent of the cases of cancer of the prostate gland in men who consume more than two daily servings of milk."[329]

Approximately 5 per cent of cancers among men would come from large consumers of dairy products. The cells would then be confused and errors may occur in the duplication of its DNA. The cells would transform into a tumor in the following manner: "Elevation of the lactic acid in the cells leads to a proliferation of cells which will not reach their maturity (the quantity destroyed the quality) and would be unable to capture the oxygen and to eliminate the waste."[330]

Psychiatric pathologies, malformations, cancers in children exposed to synthetic hormones would be compounded if they are associated with the quantities of synthetic estrogen or progesterone. Is it that the use of contraceptive pills could cause of cancers in the child who is born to the result of the termination of this medication even several years later?

"This spontaneous cohort represents an example Grandeur nature of the impact neurodéveloppemental of synthetic hormones on the emergence of behavioral disorders in humans."[331] We know that hormones act on the personality and behavior of the people. We only have to think of all the mood swings related to the crisis of adolescence, and premenstrual syndrome which has long been perceived by the medical system as a psychiatric illness. The Bodybuilders who inject steroids can become violent and powerless. It is not surprising to find that behavior disorders can therefore be linked to meat and dairy products which would be packed with hormones.

A recipe very secret

It would also have been found traces of pesticides, fertilizers and dioxin in the dairy products. The meat of beef in Canada can contain carcinogenic hormones and endocrine regulators in addition of antibiotics. Even if people make us believe that there is not in Quebec, a lot of meat would come from the western provinces or the United States. The hormones would even be used as a food additive and find themselves in the meat.

"Are Also found in the milk of pest control residues, anti-inflammatory, pesticides and aflatoxins strongly carcinogenic."[332] traces of anti-inflammatory drugs would also have been found in the milk of ibuprofen. In Europe, a glass of milk can contain up to 20 chemicals including analgesics and fungicides. "For a traditional breeding, is found in the milk of traces of vaccines, hormones and drugs used to treat the cows as well as chemical pollutants in their food."[333]

The food pollution

The milk, chicken meat, pork and beef in some countries in Europe have been suspected to contain dioxin. Dioxin is a persistent pollutant in the environment which may eventually find themselves in our plates. It comes from the pulp and paper industries and the combustion of plastics of Waste incinerators including some from of the releases of hospitals. It is removal on the plants that the animals eat. It accumulates mainly in fat such as the yellow of eggs, milk and animal fat.

Dioxins are highly toxic and can cause problems in the reproduction, development, harming the immune system, interfere with the hormonal system and cause cancers. There is the highest concentrations in some soils, sediments, and foods, including dairy products, meat, fish and crustaceans.[334]

The dioxin would have been found in a food additive in Europe. If certain equipment of dairy are actually made of tin, is that milk could contain traces of heavy metals. The tin is a toxic heavy metal. Without interior coating, food stored can absorb it. The tin cause of gastro-intestinal disorders.

The lies of the food industry

The traces of hormones in dairy products can lower the rate of calcium in the blood. The presence of hormones in meat and milk would prevent us to absorb nutrients and to assimilate the calcium. This would explain why some people with osteoporosis are in effect of heavy drinkers of milk. The lack of calcium would ensure that our body the draws from even its organization. The body become too acid draws on its reserves to try to restore its pH, which makes the bones porous.

In the liver, a growth hormone can lose to the body its ability to use the nutrients. Calcium is often at the decline in autistic children even if they are addicted to dairy products. The nervous system has need of calcium. Drink too much milk could therefore affect the central nervous system. The calcium in milk, Ca+, may not be absorbed since our body has need of calcium Ca++ (doubly ionized), that found 70% in the green plants. The milk has a pH acid, and the acidifying can demineralisation of the bone structures and thus provide fertile ground for the development of cancers. "Very many common foods contain in the crude state of substances that reduce or even prevent the assimilation of certain fundamental elements that they must bring us."[335]

For example, the caffeine in coffee and chocolate would prevent us to absorb the iron. The more you drink coffee and more you are tired, and more you are tired, the more you drink coffee, whereas an iron supplement will suffice to give you the true energy you need.

The calcium in the métaboliserait milk of the calcium in the body by inhibiting the uptake of magnesium. The magnesium would be much better for our OS that the calcium. The high presence of phosphorus in the milk would prevent the absorption of calcium. Our Intestines can absorb phosphorus, which would create an imbalance between the calcium and phosphorus that the excess of the latter makes it toxic. To neutralize this excess, our body would use the calcium from our bones leading to osteoporosis. The traces of heavy metals and of anti-inflammatory drugs in milk also prevent the absorption of calcium. The rate of calcium not absorbed have repercussions on the digestive enzymes. This would be among the largest consumers of dairy products that would be the highest rate of osteoporosis.

Request to pregnant women as well as to those who are breastfeeding to pay attention to what they eat and consume a lot of dairy products. Imagine all the wrongs that can make to the fetus and the baby who risk of missing essential nutrients and absorb of hormones and antibiotics to Tower of arm.

The Japanese and the Africans will not suffer or very little of osteoporosis, because they do not consume a lot.

Heat the milk would kill all the good bacteria of milk and would lose also its nutrient values, that is why vitamins D and E would be added. The calcium has need of the Vitamin D (Sun) to be absorbed and too much calcium destroys vitamin D. then, are looking for the Error! "The study has also shown that men who drink milk fortified with vitamin D may have a very low rate of this vitamin in the body. Explains this phenomenon by the fact that the large concentration of calcium in milk eliminates the vitamin D in the body."[336]

The vegetarians of 70 years and more have a greater bone density that persons carnivores much more young people. The absorption of calcium plant is done more easily. The animals do not suffer from osteoporosis because they do not drink milk all their life. The fractures are more numerous among women who drink several glasses of milk per day.

"The milk prevents the assimilation of zinc and increases our needs in vitamins A and B12."[337]

This are therefore, in addition, of nutrients in deficit in autistic children including those who are addicted to milk. Of the substances in our food prevent us to absorb the nutrients they contain.

A food death

"The proteins of milk are very indigestible for the digestive system of the man, in particular the casein. Even if we had the stomach of a calf, pasteurization and sterilization at high temperature destroys vitamins and enzymes needed for the digestion of these proteins."[338] The pasteurization would render the calcium in the insoluble milk, which would prevent us to metabolize. It would destroy also the vitamins C, B12 and B6 whose autistic children are in lack. The surplus of casein adheres and glue to the intestinal mucosa preventing the body to absorb the nutrients. What glue to intestines night in the absorption of iron leading to anemia, a disease of more and more present in children. Most of the children with autism have a deficit in iron and calcium.

The milk powder is a reconstituted milk which contains, by the heat with which he has been treaty, losses. "The problem is that the process does not eliminate only the undesirable bacteria, but also several enzymes essential for the digestion of the milk and several vitamins naturally present in milk."[339]

In addition to all the chemicals that are found in the milk, the homogenization and pasteurization would alter its molecular structure and would kill the good bacteria, these probiotics if necessary to our intestinal health. The pasteurized milk would only contain the bad bacteria that have not been destroyed by heat, which remained in a latent state after be transformed in spore, which colonizes our intestines. The pasteurization would destroy the beneficial effect of good bacteria.

The death of the good bacteria in the milk can no longer protect us from the bad bacteria in our intestines. It is risky for people who suffer from immune deficiency. The pasteurized milk would have a pH equivalent to soft drinks.

"Pasteurization and homogenization significantly impair the composition, the digestibility and the biological availability of milk."[340]

Growth hormones and other chemical products in the milk would not be destroyed by pasteurization. The pasteurized milk would promote the diabetes, because the digestive enzymes destroyed by pasteurization are forcing the pancreas to produce too much for succeed to the Digest. Of calves would be dead after bu of the pasteurized milk. The milk contains a protein that is used for the absorption of calcium by our intestines, but it would be destroyed by pasteurization.

The pasteurization of milk products would be made to preserve them longer, but this is not the case, since the pasteurized milk is would contaminate more easily. The technological treatments of the milk may change the spatial configuration of the proteins, which distorts the milk and can form compounds allergens, since the fact to unfold the chain of casein form of the bridges that link the molecules between them. The protein (casein) would be toggled by the heat. The pasteurization could therefore be responsible for allergies to the casein. While destroying its natural assets, pasteurization would also lessen the flavor real milk.

"[...] And that the homogenization, which prevents the milk to separate from the cream, could increase the risk of high level in the blood of hormones and other chemical elements that promote the onset of cancer."[341] The homogenization would increase intolerance to milk. The homogenized milk would be associated with heart disease, as the fat is maintained mixed in the milk instead of float to the surface. This process also makes the fat globules of milk smaller, which allows them to cross the intestinal barrier and who was able to trigger the lactose intolerance and allergies to the casein. It should be checked if the autism has increased at the same time that the pasteurization and homogenization of the milk cow.

Vive the bio!

The purchase of organic foods is strongly recommended, but it must be careful, because of the natural meat is not necessarily biological, and meat controlled, not more.

"The demand for milk without synthetic hormones has increased by 500 per cent in the United States since that Monsanto has introduced its rBST fare. The organic milk is the product whose sales are growing most rapidly in the sector of organic products."[342] The organic milk is less polluted and the cows living in grand air are less stressed. In addition, the milk bio would not suffer of transformation. Organic meat contains no hormones or antibiotics and the animals are fed with grains that do not contain pesticides and that are non-GM. In addition, the animals are free to go to the outside.

The raw milk would represent less of a danger that the suspect the lobbies of the industry of the pasteurized milk. The raw milk contains antibodies that we offer resistance to diseases, is less allergen, gives less of infections to the ears and sinuses, least of asthma and colds, fewer dental caries. The food is complete and rich in micronutrients, vitamin B, antioxidants, vitamins and minerals. It also contains more omega-6. It strengthens the immune system, can diminish the allergic reactions. It contains a lot of bacteria such as Lactobacilli which help us to digest the lactose.

"It contains more than 60 enzymes, some of which help the digestion of the milk itself, thus creating less work to our pancreas."[343] The risks to be sick would be higher with the pasteurized milk that the raw milk which remains a live food. The good bacteria still present in the raw milk prevent the growth of bad bacteria. The raw milk does not cause of diarrhea.

The security at any price ($)

Despite all its virtues, the raw milk is prohibited in Canada. In any way, the multinational corporations would be stronger than the government for this which is of regulations, prohibitions and permissions. Those who would dare to express themselves on the dangerousness of a product or a process are going to be hosed by the anger of the authorities which the will force to be silenced.

"Monsanto has pursued a dairy business which was committed not to sell any product containing a synthetic hormone of growth."[344] The labelling "product containing hormones" is not mandatory. The U.S. Food and Drug Administration would have approved the use of five kinds of hormones in food production.

Everywhere in the world, the use of growth hormones in livestock raises the controversy as several countries have allowed it. The use of these products, although prohibited in Europe, would be permitted in Canada and the United States.

Tests have neglected important risks. The European Commission is asking questions about the safety of the meat in Canada to the point of refuse its import.

"How to trust to researchers who do not cease to create more perverse risks and complex that so-called benefits for human health [...]. How to trust to the industries of the Agri-Food with what we know of the nutrition of the animals and fertilizer plants."[345]

Chapter 15

The Vagaries of food and the nutrient deficit

The genetic maladaptive

The Genetics would not be the only responsible for the mental illnesses. "We know that the supply can change up to 60% the expression of our genes."[346] foods are promoters of genomes, therefore they are a factor in what differentiates the peoples. The celiac disease was not genetics at the beginning, but it would be become from generation to generation, being very subtle at the beginning. The under-supply could create of brain disorders that would be irreversible in many cases, especially if it occurs at a critical period where the brain develops. The power supply has consequences on the physical, psychological and social.

Malnutrition is when the body does not get the nutrients it needs. The nutrient deficit has not always report with the quantity of food available and gulped down. Approximately 800 million people suffer from malnutrition everywhere in the world and 25 000 people die of under-nutrition each year, of which only 17 per cent come from the under-developed countries.

We are attracted by the foods that cause us the most wrong

Children have more and more food whims, which contributes to nutrient deficiencies. Do not want to eat that macaroni and cheese to the three meals of the day leaves something to be desired. The child is in need of a menu more balanced.

If you do not offer to the child a food which has the same color, the same texture and taste the same as that which gives it a certain effect, it will refuse to eat during a certain period, because the withdrawal of this drug seems difficult and it will seek to manipulate its parents. But a child will not die of hunger. If the food the fact suffer, the child may prefer to consume foods that are similar to what he already knows, refusing to taste new dishes, because it is more secure for him. These children would have been marked by the pain. They will always have the vagaries food, because their brains would have recorded that eating = suffer. It will be difficult to unschedule. The food has made them live very bad experiences. Be difficult with food may lead to the development of chronic diseases.

If a child with autism or ADHD is especially attracted by foods that contain gluten and casein, it is because he loves the sensations that it provides. An actress has already said on TV that her son is a "autism happy". Certainly, as said so well a popular expression: "It is frozen as a ball!" It is a bit like an alcoholic. He knows that he is going to be sick with headaches and stomach, but this does not prevent the drink, because the mental sensations pleasant OUTWEIGH THE INCONVENIENCE physical.

Dependencies are manifested by a food sensitivity, which fact that people are attracted by these foods because the body governs the stress caused by these products by secreting a substance to protect us, which causes in us a habituation.

"And you can become addicted to these drugs that our body manufactures."[347] This process would explain why the cereals and dairy products are the foods most consumed in our western civilization. This would explain in part the vagaries food, because these foods act as drugs: "The more you in consumed, and more you want!" These molecules of proteins, called "peptides", travel in the blood from a porous intestine up to the brain where they cause of neurological disorders such as would some derived from opium. Give the gluten or casein to a child who is intolerant, it is the same thing as the prick with heroin. The gluten and casein would be the "cocaine" of the power supply. The regime CSMS fact appear of withdrawal symptoms powerful, the same as those of a drug addict. The child has less food whims and it is more attracted to other foods offering him a menu more varied and nutritious when the regime SGSCSS (without gluten, without casein and without soy) is in place and maintained.

Of the opium in my plate

The casein and gluten are foods containing opioid peptides. Opioid intoxication can cause autistic traits. The autism is connected to an excess of opiates in the brain. We can also compare their effect to morphine. "The prolonged exposure to these peptides opiates could have many effects on the brain in growth of the young child, as with any other narcotic."[348] The presence of peptides opiates has been discovered also in the urine of hyperactive children.

The work of Dohan, Reichelt, Shattock, CADE as well as other researchers have highlighted the high rates of peptides of the gluten and casein - called glutamorphine and casomorphines - in the urine of patients suffering from autism, schizophrenia, psychosis, depression, hyperactivity with attention deficit as well as in some cases of diseases Autoimmune disorders.[349]

These opioid peptides saturate the brain and inhibit the social behavior as well as the development of the language, disrupt the hormones which serotonin which has an impact on sleep disorders and on the impulsive reactions, as well as on the difficulties of adaptation. The molecule of gluten so resembles an opiate that it would on the receptors of these peptides, which influence the entire nervous system.

All those who love the milk, cheese, bread and pastries should ask themselves questions. Approximately 30% of adults would be intolerant to gluten and only 10% could.

On the biological plan, we are not made to eat as we do. Our organization is not accustomed and our system has not even had the time to adapt. We are not of livestock to feed us with as much grain products in all its forms: pizzas, pasta, breads, pastries. It is not surprising that several people develop an intolerance to gluten with the time. There are dairy products, wheat and soybeans in almost everything we eat: processed food products, pre-cooked dishes, sauces and other accompaniments. There has been too rapid changes in our modern diet. We do not eat enough fruit and vegetables.

At the beginning, the gluten presents symptoms very subtle often categorized as a psychiatric disorder. Celiac disease is silent, sneaky, underhanded, and unpredictable: it has caused a lot of damage before to be discovered. The symptoms vary from one person to another, passing by the agitation or depression, backaches, digestive disorders, headaches and nasal congestion. Intolerance to gluten cause of stunted growth and disrupts the functioning of the brain. Dyslexia and the school problems may be due to intolerance to gluten, even that of sleep disorders and the lack of confidence in itself. The gluten disrupts the socialization, affectivity and the programming. "Fed to gluten, the rat loses its faculties of learning, the Cat adopts a strange behavior, kittens, puppies and the chicks do not cry at weaning."[350]

And yet, there is in the commercial food for our pets. It nourishes therefore carnivores with cereal grains such as corn, wheat and rice. Yet, I have never seen them devour a field of grasses. There is even the gluten in the food of some fish aquarium.

New chronic diseases are related to the intolerance to gluten. The gluten affects the position of neurons in a brain in full development. There is a relation between the Schizophrenia and the consumption of cereals. The opioid peptides, to force to move easily across the barrier hemato-meningeal, can increase the permeability of the latter to the force of the bomb. It would be a form of porosity similar to that of the intestinal mucosa. A saturation of receptors occurs. The progressive malfunction comes from the inhibition of the development of the brain by the accumulation of opiate peptides. The gluten would contain 16 molecules opioids. The development of mental and behavioral disorders is favored by the accumulation of neurons. Autism may well be the form the most chronicle of the celiac disease. The gluten promotes the development of degenerative diseases of the nervous system. Here is everything that can cause a intoxication in gluten:

Some examples: school problems, dyspraxia, dyslexia, attention deficit and conduct disorder, hypo and hyperactivity, relational problems, violence, various types of autism (with or without language), disorders of the convulsive involuntary (tics), obsessive-compulsive disorders (OCD), self-mutilation, sleep disturbance, chronic fatigue, illness of the intestine (bloating, constipation, disease of the intestine), schizophrenia, etc.[351]

We can have a sensitivity to gluten without be celiac. As well, there is the presence of the peptides of gluten, and often also of casein, in the urine of individuals with schizophrenia, epilepsy, of people with autism and hyperactive. However, these intolerances are unknown, of people with the disease.

"A scheme of this type [CSMS] is also proposed by the Doctor Jean Seignalet, Doctor Immunologist in the hospital St. Eloi of Montpellier, now deceased, to mitigate the symptoms of rheumatoid and Crohn's disease ."[352]

The allergy to gluten contributes to an increase in health problems, because it damages the intestines, destroyed the digestive enzymes and lowers the defense mechanisms. The power supply is an environmental impact which acts on the immune system.

"But as the peptides (GC) are very similar to those which constitute some of our fabrics, this disease can degenerate into autoimmune disease in which our own immune system to attack the liver or the nervous system, or the intestinal wall (celiac disease) or the brain."[353]

The gluten-free diet helps the learning difficulties, the dysphasia, the dyspraxia and dyslexia. The improvement with the change in food has place on plans cognitive and behavioral. Among the people with Parkinson's Disease, 60% reveal themselves to be intolerant to gluten.

The medical system does not find solutions to serious diseases, then that by closing the porous permeability of the intestine, well of disorders are reportedly conceal. Because of the Greater intestinal permeability, people with autism are the most sensitive to these foods which eventually be very intoxicated. The choice of our diet has an impact on our health and on the development of new chronic diseases and degenerating. "In England, Dr. Natasha Campbelle McGridge, neurologist, has made the link between the pathologies of the intestine permeable and of the brain (autism, dyslexia, dyspraxia, dysphasia, disturbance in attention, depression)."[354]

The intestine is often red and damaged. During the Second World War, the rate of autism would have decreased because the people in the short of wheat have eaten more of potatoes. Since 20 years, autism and hyperactivity have not ceased to grow as well as the juvenile schizophrenia. During 50 years, wheat would have suffered up to 50 transformations and changes, and we had that two generations for us to live with it. The current wheats have two times more gluten than the former. The intestine is normally impervious to undesirable substances that it eliminates by the stool, but in the case of a intestinal hyperperméabilité, substances pass through the intestinal wall and are found in the blood and the lymphatic system to go to remove to the brain, or the joints or the organs and create rheumatic diseases, neurological or digestive tract, since not everyone reacts the same way to this intolerance. The difference between a child TED and a child ADHD would then depend on the intestinal porosity. The hyperactivity would have increased by 700 per cent during the last decade.

"A malfunction of metabolism prevents the disintegration of some proteins (including casein present in the milk), which could then cause disorders of behavior, including a disorder of the deficit for the attention of the hyperactivity (ADHD)."[355]

There is a link between hyperactivity and attention deficit with autism since an autistic child also suffers from hyperactivity and attention deficit. Therefore, the ADHD would be a less severe form of autism and could be part of the same family. In both cases, there is a difficulty to assimilate or metabolize Vitamin B12. The B vitamins are metabolized by the intestinal system when it is in good health and that its flora has not been damaged or destabilized. The imbalance of the intestinal flora plays a role in ADHD. The hyperactive children have a lack of iron, which creates the link with the intolerance to gluten.

Peoples such as the Italians who consume a lot of gluten with pasta, pizza and bread would be among those who there would have the highest rate of autism. The gluten cause a delay of growth by the intestinal lesions that it product. Intolerant people to gluten must also avoid dairy products.

"In fact, intolerance to gluten is almost always a celiac disease that destroys the villi of the intestine in its upper part, which hinders or prevents the production of lactase (digestive enzyme) and which causes the lactose intolerance ."[356]

Therefore, the allergy to the casein is also caused by the gluten; that is why, in the results of analysis of peptides in the urine, a positive result in a automatically suggests the withdrawal of the two. Intolerance to gluten and casein can cause a dysbiose which is an imbalance of the intestinal flora. The intestines select certain types of bacteria in our intestines some of which are neurotoxicantes. The immune system is overreacting to the molecules too often encountered in producing a large quantity of antibodies that clog the blood.

"Although this plan is controversial within the medical community, some physicians make the promotion for children with autism. The journalist Thierry Sauccar denounces an operation of lobbying."[357] The grain products and dairy products represent very much for the economy, then it should especially not that people cease to consume, and even if it makes them sick, this is not serious, they will be packed with pills very profitable also for the industry.

The children more intoxicated will go up to make seizures because the opioids have properties seizures, which explains the small poorly among the students of Primary: those who often fall into the moon.

The rituals and stereotypes are for children of the behaviors that the secure, because their nervous system would be surstimulé, which explains their emotional sensitivity and sensory. Did you know that one of the small data pills to children ADHD contains a dye, whose yellow, which itself would cause of hyperactivity?

The medical tests to detect the celiac disease or intolerance to gluten are effective only in the most serious situations where there has been heavy damage, otherwise the result of the test may be falsely negative, even when there is a sensitivity to gluten. Instead of doing the tests unreliable, remove the gluten from your supply of three weeks to three months and you will see if you go better.

The most famous food intolerance is that lactose which would affect 75 per cent of the present world population. If the milk can cause of eczema and the hives, then what is it used to prescribe to the soothing creams when the problem comes from the inside?

Another problem with the allergies caused by vaccines is the presence of albumin in the gluten which would be similar to the albumin of animal used in the manufacture of some vaccines. Given that we do not eat through the skin of the arm, the immune system would develop antibodies against all kinds of albumin, which can be another cause in the development of intolerance to gluten.

The casein would address more specifically to the part of the brain responsible for the development of the language; that is why our son is put to speak when we have removed the dairy products (and the soybean) of its power. The peptides of the Soybean resemble those of the casein and this would be one of the reasons for which the soybean also influence the development of the language. The Soybean is part of the power supply Japanese and Chinese and it arrived too quickly and in too large quantities in our western menu. "Its allergenicity is conferred by several distinct proteins. The hypersensitivity to one of these proteins is sufficient to develop an allergy to soy. In some cases, the children who are allergic to cow milk fed with soy milk may develop a hypersensitivity."[358]

The soy milk cannot therefore replace the cow milk. The delays and disorders of the language (which are live speech therapists) would have increased in the same time that the development of the agri-food industry, and the result of the many ads surrounding the Dairy Products. But, again, people will say that it is only a coincidence. This term would explain everything but does not excuse everything. At its therapy with a speech therapist for more than a year and a half, my son has learned that two or three new words; it makes very expensive the syllable to $90 an hour once a week.

The system of education would not be the promotion of the health of young people, but rather that of the pharmaceutical industry when stakeholders require the parents, to the force of pressure, threats and blackmail, to give Ritalin to children while they close their eyes on the recent discoveries. Imagine Berlingots of milk in the classes of language disorders. Ironic, is it not? It gives them a ripe fruit, CRU, fresh and organic to the place. After having worked as a teacher for nearly 12 years in primary, I had the time to see the changes among my students after the morning snack. Some complained of headaches and stomach. I have even heard of teachers say that dairy products disrupt the brain of some children, but all continued to give them. However I am not the only one to have mentioned. I even sent a press release to the concerned school boards for the notify with a copy of the article, and some have told me that they follow the recommendations of the Canadian Food Guide which also must be handled by the agri-food industry. Me, I personally believe that the Ritalin helps more the teacher that the child itself, since this does not solve the problem at the source.

And yet, there is something in the milk which prevents children to speak. When I speak of the Directorates to school, I am stare as if I was a extraterrestrial. I even displayed in the room of the teachers last year another article in the newspaper of Montreal from 7 July 2009 WHO announces in title: "autism may heal", and someone, I strongly suspect the director, has ripped off. It is necessary that the people remain in ignorance; C is the best way to handle. It is misinformation.

Today, the cow does not just eating hay or of the fresh grass. It is nourished with genetically modified cereals that have pushed with toxic chemicals, in addition to receiving vaccines containing heavy metals, antibiotics and hormones. Traces of all this can be found in the milk that one gives joyfully to drink to children in firmly believing that this is good for them. Why? Because we have grown up with this mentality.

Treason or manipulation?

"The dairy industry is heard with restaurants of fast preparation to add more cheese to their food to trigger our rage of cheese."[359]

Why, according to you, the pizza is it so popular? Because that is the 100% gluten and casein. And is there about the small baskets of fresh bread placed at our disposal on the table of restaurants in our arrival?

Cross-contamination

In some food processing industries, the equipment can be poorly cleaned and disinfected incorrectly, which could cause cross-contamination. This contamination has place when of gluten-free foods are produced in factories where the manufacture of other products which contain gluten. Just traces of gluten in a product or on the dishes of the same that the utensils may be harmful.

The views are very controversial about the gluten in the oats. Some say that the oats in contains and others argue the contrary. Regardless, the two clans have reason. The oats is contaminated by the wheat with the rotation of crops and with agricultural equipment used.

"The cross-contamination is the process by which a Food without gluten lost this status because it comes into contact with something which is not without gluten."[360] There would be no gliadin (gluten) in oats, except that its molecule, the avenin, is very similar. It can, therefore, by its likeness, be considered by the Organization as of the gluten, just as the molecule of the soybean that looks so to that of casein that it can cause the same problems. An intolerance to a automatically causes the sensitivity to the other. The similarity between the gliadin and the avenin is so noticeable that it is strongly recommended to people with celiac disease or those who are intolerant to gluten to try to consume oats that under medical supervision to see if the body would accept.

A similar problem also happens with corn, which explains why several autistic children or persons intolerant gluten develop such an allergy. The different mutations in the evolution of the Corn makes this species present very different from the existing one and consumed thousands of years ago, which risk of developing an allergy.

Diseases of the food

The obsession for food would come from a sub-Power or its effects. "Of the obsessions and compulsions related to food may be caused or exacerbated by malnutrition."[361]

The sub-Power and the anorexia create of depressive states. Mental disorders are derived from genetic factors, biological and environmental factors. Nutrition therefore has an impact on mental health. "The undernourished individuals become irritable, depressive, tired."[362]

The sensitivity to noise, which is a symptom, autism is a consequence psychological an under-supply. Malnutrition causes the shame and the downturn on itself, and this, not just because of the appearance. It also causes of sleep disorders, another of the autistic symptoms. The deficiencies make the body more vulnerable to infections, that is why the depressed people are more prone to colds and flu. The resistance to infections depends on the nutrition, and each infection influence the supply since we have less hungry when we are sick.

Of Mental illnesses such as anorexia and bulimia are indeed an eating disorder. Therefore, the supply acts on the brain and behavior. Of anomalies at neurotransmitters influence the mood and the appetite. Of nutrient deficiencies can therefore develop the vagaries of food, and vice versa; this is not because it eats a lot that we eat well. The modernization pushes us to eating improperly. In addition, the bread, pastries and fat, such as dairy products, are the foods that are more fattening. Then, persons suffering from a surplus of weight should ask themselves if they are not addicted to these foods.

Hard as iron

Dietary deficiencies can cause disorders of health physical and mental. A decrease of essential proteins, either because they are poorly digested or not well assimilated, causes major malfunctions and multiple-including a retardation of growth and a decline of the faculties of the immune system. The brain lack of vitamins, good essential fats, proteins and minerals and well digested. A lack in amino acids prevents the Agency to renew its proteins and this lack can cause thyroid disorders including obesity, diabetes, asthma, renal impairment as well as osteoarthritis.

According to a UNICEF report in 2004: "The iron deficiency among infants 6 to 24 months affect the mental development. Iodine deficiency have made back the intellectual capacity. The lack of vitamin A causes the death of a thousand children each year."[363] The lack of iron can cause the death of 60 000 women during childbirth or during pregnancy. The Sub-power supply has caused 58% of the Mortality in 2006, which is equivalent to 36 million people who died of hunger or diseases related to the nutrient deficiency. Eating disorders occur in countries in full development.

The nutrient deficiencies are present also in the most industrialized countries. Eat just or often of grain products and dairy products leads to a nutrient imbalance since food badly digested cannot be assimilated.

The poisoning in gluten is caused by the presence of heavy metals including mercury. It is a genetic predisposition triggered by an environmental impact. Of the poisonings to heavy metals cause an intestinal permeability, and thus of food intolerances.

The vaccines to thimerosal or containing aluminum could be of the triggers of the celiac disease and other forms of intoxication to gluten. The people who are likely to become allergic to gluten possess on the genetic map of the sensors that allow them unfortunately to fix heavy metals. It is the association between the heavy metals, the gluten and casein which sometimes cause problem.

"And accumulate in the body, the heavy metals have an inhibitory action on the peptidases, a family of enzymes intended for the degradation of a set of dietary proteins."[364]

It is a dysregulation of the enzyme system which cause the intolerance to gluten. The degradation of certain enzymes leads to a failure of the metabolism. The absence of protein degradation flooded the blood which may obstruct a good blood circulation. Nurses say they have difficulty in taking blood samples to children with autism. Children with a disorder of behavior have a deficiency in peptidases (enzymes). The hyperactivity that derives from among children may go up to the depression in adults.

Food badly digested become allergens. Then, if you acknowledge the food in your stool: pieces of corn, carrots, nuts or salad, is that you should not eat, because it will not give you nothing.

Measles and hunger

Feed well help us to fight infections. The measles virus is dangerous and deadly only in the under-developed countries because the people who are suffering from malnutrition are powerless before an infection. It is a nutrient deficit which makes measles if virulent. If the rate of autism has increased rapidly in the poor countries after a massive vaccination, is that there is a link between the vaccine of measles and malnutrition. Poor nutrition is part of malnutrition because the overconsumption of food of the type fast food contributes to a nutrient deficit, even that the fact to be addicted to the one or two categories of foods. Malnutrition is due to a nutrient deficiency, and it also exists in countries highly developed. Here, in the most industrialized countries, the nutrient deficit is caused by intolerance to gluten. Therefore, I gather that in principle the measles vaccine should not be given to children who suffer from malnutrition.

It would be wiser to do tests in the level of iron to a child before the vaccinated to ensure that it can support the vaccine, in the same way that is done before a blood donation. It seems to me that this is not so complicated. Nobody has thought about it in the medical field or nobody bothered to think about it. And it is me, a single mom who comes to make this great medical discovery by putting all the pieces of the puzzle together.

The triggering of the genetic predisposition to celiac disease by the MMR vaccine would explain why this are not all children who become with Autism or ADHD after this vaccine, because the measles virus affects only the children who suffer from malnutrition or who are inclined to develop a nutrient deficit of any kind such as anemia and celiac disease. Consume too much of cereals can be detrimental to the immunization of vaccines injected. The lack of good protein cause of stunted growth, especially when they are not digested and assimilated. Malnutrition can be also characterized by excessive consumption and inadequate protein. Other unlucky children would develop with time the diabetes or cancer linked to a immuno-reaction weakened or reversed.

The aluminum in vaccines is also lower the level of iron. The iron is important for red blood cells and the functions of certain enzymes. The anemia, thus caused, brings a deficiency in essential nutrients to the cells whose immune system has greatly need during a vaccination. She brings a reduction of intellectual and physical abilities, less resistance to infections and disturbances in the growth. The different forms of autism have a link with the different kinds of poisoning to gluten, which depend on the severity of the Intestinal porosity. Give the iron can help a child, for as much as the gluten and casein are deleted; otherwise, the iron may not be absorbed.

There is a link between malnutrition and infectious disease. An immune system improperly nourished cannot carry out its work. "Infections will worsen the malnutrition and poor nutrition accentuates the severity of infectious diseases."[365] The AIDS leads to a form of malnutrition, because the secondary infections cause an improper assimilation of nutrients. Tuberculosis is also assimilated to the leanness. Bacterial infections cause a loss of nitrogen in the body; and c is one of the ways in which a infection affects the nutritional status. The infections decrease the appetite. It may be therefore that vaccines cause a difficulty to assimilate nutrients that would help the immune system to fight them. It seems to me that it is logical.

A gastroenteritis creates a nutrient slump. The diarrhea reduces the absorption of nutrients, and vaccines as the MMR vaccine can cause diarrhea.

Of the children who suffer from an infection as a result of diarrhea are not able to manufacture of antibodies. Diarrhea can cause irreversible damage to the brain. Therefore, malnutrition can cause mental infirmities. The MMR vaccine would cause of diarrhea. And doctors will say to parents not to do if their baby has diarrhea after a vaccine. And even if it lasts for two years, they find this "normal" then that it is "fatal".

"In the same way, children suffering from protein-energy malnutrition have an immune reaction faulty when their inoculates the vaccine."[366]

The doctors would be wrong to say that the Vaccines strengthen the immune system. Therefore, viruses and bacteria, they are injected or not, cause a weakening of the immune system especially in a body to the taken with a nutrient deficit of some kind, because this deficit is often caused by the infection itself.

"These examples show how diseases such as measles, respiratory infections of tracks high and gastro-intestinal infections can contribute to the development of the malnutrition."[367]

Physical and mental health problems exist among the homeless people who suffer from nutritional deficiencies often caused by the invasion of parasites. There is a relationship between the intestinal parasites, diarrhea, nutrition and the measles virus. Parasites cause debilitating diseases; other cause intestinal hemorrhage, which prevents the proteins to be well digested and the iron to be absorbed. Parasites live in the intestines of 600 million people in the world. The parasites, just as the yeasts to Candida, cause a malnutrition since these sales bugs feed on what we eat. The yeasts prevent the absorption of nutrients. To get rid of these parasites gives impact on the physical and psychological development. An infection can cause a nutrient deficit. For example, a parasite of fish loves the vitamin B12 creating a deficiency in its host.

If measles is fatal only in the poor countries suffering from malnutrition, it is mainly because of the presence of a parasite with which the virus would team. And advertising campaigns we are afraid with this disease just to sell their vaccine since to be fatal in the developed countries, it must be that the child has already a precarious state of health. Here, the virus against measles has as an ally the Candida. Therefore, a child who has a yeast infection may respond poorly to the vaccine for measles, while the proliferation of Candida is favored by the taking of antibiotics, which proves once again the link between vaccines and antibiotics in the development of autism.

The virus is also serve the assistance of yeasts and heavy metals to build shelters in order to develop their virulence by clinging to a intestinal mucosa damaged which serves as their refuge for not

215

getting caught by the antibodies. That is why a large quantity of measles antibody was allegedly found in the intestines of autistic children by Dr. Wakefield.

The measles virus can cause blindness.

"The exact mechanism of this relationship of cause and effect is not established, but it is likely that many of the infections have for consequence to reduce the absorption of vitamin A."[368]

This explains why several children have an eye that ladle after a vaccine and that the problem with the strabismus may be adjusted with vitamin A supplements, including several children with autism are deficient. Is it that the measles vaccine could thus make blind children?

"Measles can also be responsible for the deficiency in vitamin A."[369] a vitamin A supplement can also help to go through the disease of the measles, instead of cripple thousands of children with vaccines. The sequelae are of psychological orders, governmental and social.

The merry Three Musketeers

Vaccines have as allies the heavy metals to cause damage to the intestines and enzymes of digestion. This are the toxic metals present in the vaccines that would help the virus to intervene through to the food deficit, and it is often a combination of the two that creates the impact. They have also as third partner yeasts, which create a first nutrient deficit. The association between the heavy metals, gluten and yeast is indestructible.

The Mercure alter in the first place the intestinal wall which opens the path to the gluten, and aluminum aid to the nutrient deficit by lowering the iron. The heavy metals cover Viruses and thus protects against the action of the immune system. The vaccines would therefore be one of the largest medical errors in the history of humanity. In addition, it does not help the immune system in feeding the yeasts of what they prefer: the starchy foods and dairy products.

An alteration of the blood-brain barrier may also, just as the intestinal mucosa, be caused by an imbalance of the enzyme. The judgments of the language can therefore be caused by viruses including those of vaccines in contact with the opioid peptides of the brain, because they are used for protein to cross the barrier. The aluminum is not blocking just the absorption of iron, but also access to the serotonin. Because children with autism have a disability in serotonin, it is that the aluminum, including one of the vaccines, plays a role in the onset of autism.

216

Autism may well be part of diseases of malnutrition in link with a any intoxication.

The Health Foundations has been handed back to the children who have followed the diet without gluten or casein, and sometimes even without Soybean Corn or if they have followed, in addition to a chelation and if they have taken appropriate supplements to their personal condition while leading a fight against the intestinal yeasts. The everything is done before their body and especially their brains have suffered too much irreparable damage because the cells of the brain are not replaced.

A brain hungry and thirsty

A decline of elements necessary does not help the body to function well. How can he find all the resources to fight infections, toxins, heavy metals as well as pollutants from the air and the power supply? The lack of an essential element and the presence of foreign elements in the brain affect the operation of neurotransmitters.

If the nutrient deficiencies can cause the baldness because the hair lack of micronutrients necessary for their health, I dare suggest that if the nutrients does not go to the hair roots, they therefore cannot go to the brain.

A meal is rich in carbohydrates acts on amino acids and on the production of serotonin: this would be at the base of the brain nutrition.

A deficit maternal nutrient affects the distribution of the elements essential to the fetus, which can lead to cognitive disorders and behavior problems with neurological impairment who could become obvious. To work well, our neurons have need of energy. The brain has need of oxygen that is transported by the blood, which contains 80% of water. During a dehydration, the blood becomes thicker and carries less of nutrients and oxygen to the brain. "A slight deficit in water is enough to bring down our brain performance."[370]

The toxins are evacuated by the urine, but to urinate, it must drink a lot. Dehydration can raise the acidity of the body creating the oxidation that degrades the cells including those of the brain. Therefore, all acidic foods have an impact on the brain, and dairy and cereal products are part of acidic foods or can leave traces of acidity. The brain is one of the bodies that has the most in need of water, oxygen, nutrients and good fats. It must therefore meet the needs of the brain and the nervous system. By lack of essential elements, the brain declines and between In a phase of degeneration that can lead to the senility.

The brain, like all the other organs and system of the body, may not work well if it is poorly fed. The iron supports the activities of neurotransmitters. Forty nutrients involved in brain functions. A shortage of the enzyme could lead to a nutrient deficit. When a person has a disability in enzymes as most of the children with autism, a nutrient can accumulate and become toxic because the organization cannot metabolize; that is why supplements with help enzyme in the absorption and use by the body of vitamins, minerals and essential fat. The diseases known up to now as mental disorders can be treated by the taking of digestive enzymes. Several health problems in North America, including neurological disorders, are related to problems of digestion.

"For that nutrients are metabolized and nourish the cells of the body, all the enzymes must perform their functions. In short, the nutrients provided by the power supply must undergo several transformations to be properly used by the cells."[371]

This is not too many supplements that can do harm to certain bodies, but the lack of enzymes to assimilate. If one of the steps in the metabolism is blocked, an accumulation of toxic elements follows. It must be an adequate intake between digestive enzymes and nutritious foods and supplements, but the balance is not always easy to find. This are the enzymes which allow us to draw the greatest nutritional value of our food, because they allow us to digest well and help our body to well assimilate them. By lack of iron, the blood is no longer enough oxygen and the cells lack of oxygen and die, which because of the porosity to membranes which have the function of protecting us.

"The Iron is essential to many proteins and enzymes of our Organization. This is particularly a compound essential to the haemoglobin, a protein used by red blood cells to carry oxygen."[372] An autoimmune disease can go up to destroy its own red blood cells. The autism would be a metabolic disease. Cellular membranes attacked by the autoimmune disease pass the free radicals that bombard its kernel and lead to errors in the Cellular duplications, which could result in chronic complications. The essential fats, when they are well absorbed, protect this membrane, which protects the genetic material of its nucleus.

In addition, the enzymes are necessary to repair cells, organs and tissues, to provide energy to the cells so that they do not die, to stimulate the brain and to digest the food. They help to the heart beats, to heal the wounds, to bind the iron to the red blood cells and to transform the phosphorus in the bony parts.

There is more enzymes in raw foods which have a function of prédigestion once ingested before our own enzymes are involved. Eat raw, therefore Foods Alive, contributes to a better digestion and therefore to a better assimilation of what they contain. The cooked food processed contain very little of enzymes or not at all. The decline in the rate of enzymes available provides less resistance to infections. Raw foods are antioxidants that protect against cancer. Therefore, even the taking of enzymes may help to combat cancer.

A lack of enzymes can make us sick and shorten our life. Food badly digested can rot and cause of putrefaction with an accumulation of waste in our intestines. In decomposing, these faecal matter produce toxins and bacteria which eventually cross the blood system across the intestines in the place of the nutrients absorption is blocked by their deposits. Take enzymes can help to eliminate toxins.

Organic foods have more nutritional value. However, they are more expensive because they are difficult to cultivate and to find. If all the world were to eat organic products, this would lower their prices and increase their availability.

A nutrient deficit in protein is caused by the indigestabilité of certain animal proteins (casein) and plants (gluten). This deficit because of the impact on the functioning of all systems of the body. The lack of protein and the effect opiate of some of them would cause delays of growth and of development disorders. Some children with autism and ADHD take of enzymes as supplements to help them and they are better.

My engine is in need of an oil change

Omega-3 act as a lubricant allowing to neurons to function better. The lack of good fat night at the transmission between the cells of the brain. "The tests suggest that the imbalances or shortcomings in the unsaturated fatty acids (HUFA) can cause learning disabilities or behavior including ADHD, dyslexia, dysphasia."[373]

If the intestines are damaged, if the intestinal mucosa is overloaded, if the intestinal villi are destroyed, the fat can not be well absorbed. Omega-3 fatty acids are essential for the functioning of the brain, hormonal, inflammatory and circulatory. They also have properties anti-allergic. The DHA plays a role in the mobility of the sperm, the development of the retina and the brain. A deficit in good fats can therefore cause disturbances of vision. It also causes a disruption of the structures of the cell membranes, which may damage them.

"In effect, they maintain the integrity of cell membranes, generate energy, produce hormones, help the assimilation of vitamins and minerals as well as the normal functioning of the brain, the nervous system and the eyes."[374]

This lack disrupts the enzymatic activities of the brain, the transfer of information interneurons, which disrupts nerve transmission. A lack of good fat, what is called "good cholesterol", cause a sensitivity to light, which is often present in most of the children with autism because the liver overburdened with toxins has not managed to transform the good fats in good cholesterol. A deficiency causes of learning difficulties, affects the behavior, hormones and emotions. of omega oils greatly assist children who have problems in school. Essential fatty acids are necessary to the functioning of the nervous system. The brain is composed of 40 to 60% of fat.

Essential fatty acids (good cholesterol) reduce hypertension, relieve arthritis, are used antioxidants, Font Decrease the growth of cancerous tumors, and help combat the bad cholesterol, skin diseases, mental disorders and hormone levels.

"The two fatty acids contained in fish oils considerably improve the manic-depressive psychosis. The people suffering of aggressiveness, dementia, Alzheimer's and attention deficit disorders with hyperactivity are deficient in EPA and DHA."[375]

Consume bad fats affects the operation of the cellular structure. The Good fats contribute to the structuring of the cellular membranes, which form a barrier against infections and harmful substances. There is the good and the bad cholesterol. The Good fats which are not absorbed create a deficit in good cholesterol which the brain has both need. The Cholesterol is indispensable to life, because it plays an essential role in the synthesis of hormones and is at the origin of the components of cellular membranes. Several essential hormones are produced from the good cholesterol, and hormones interfere in the development of neurons. This would explain why girls are generally better than boys at school.

The development of the brain can be disrupted by a lack of good cholesterol (essential fatty acids), which can cause a intellectual deficit. Some children with autism have a disability in cholesterol.

The Liver ensures the synthesis of cholesterol according to the food source in bold. It is the liver which guarantees a cholesterol necessary and normal, to the extent that it works well and that it is not disturbed by the sugar and bad fats. A qualified liver of lazy will produce an excess of cholesterol. Most of the children with autism have a malfunction of the liver. Foods do not contain really of cholesterol as such since the majority of cholesterol is produced by our body from the fat in the diet. Approximately 20% of the cholesterol comes from food and 80% is produced by the liver. The digestion and assimilation of vitamins and fats would be impossible without cholesterol. Therefore, those who suffer a decrease in good cholesterol may also suffer a nutrient deficit.

"Cholesterol thus favors the permeability of the cell and allows him to breathe and feed well."[376]

It is used to the growth and repair of cells. It is therefore essential to the cellular life. A bad absorption of essential fats, often caused by the deficit in enzymes, can contribute to a intestinal porosity. Of the people who have taken drugs lipid lowering have had serious health problems, because cholesterol is a component of myelin in the brain. Of children with autism who have a deficit in cholesterol have for the most part a myelin that has lost its sealing. A bad state of the myelin sheath could lead to multiple sclerosis. The pollutants such as gases and heavy metals make this matrix of increasingly thin. The health of the brain depends upon its protection. Therefore, the saturated fat may attack the brain. When there is too much bad fats in our diet, the brain suffers as it is the body which contains the most fat. The bad fats disrupt the fluidity of neurons. The Good fats (good cholesterol) helps in the assimilation of vitamins B, C and E, which are important for the brain.

"Researchers now suspect that conventional treatments lipid lowering could have a link with Alzheimer's Disease."[377]

It is necessary to choose the right foods in order to produce good cholesterol. The polyunsaturated oils are rich in fatty acids and help to the dissolution of the bad cholesterol which the oil of fish and duck. The oils of evening primrose, borage, flax, sesame and olive oil are very good. Most of the good cholesterol is a vegetable source. The bad cholesterol is most of the time of animal source, except with respect to fish and poultry. The bad saturated fat and trans fat present in our diet do increase the rate of bad cholesterol. The good cholesterol decreases the presence of bad cholesterol in the blood, but the presence of bad cholesterol fact diminish the presence of the good cholesterol. Too many bad cholesterol is harmful; not enough good cholesterol is dangerous.

The bad cholesterol would retain the toxins in us since fats retain toxins. Then, the bad cholesterol would be detrimental to the detoxification. Avoid the bad cholesterol would help our body to get rid of toxins. That is why the former were as many therapeutic virtues in olive oil (good cholesterol).

Even the obese people would be more poisoned than the others. The lack in essential nutrients pushes people to cravings. If an obese person increased the presence of good cholesterol, it would be less scope to the fatty foods. It is one of the things which would enable him to lose weight. The overweight would be linked to an imbalance in serotonin which is a neurotransmitter. Serotonin would play a role in the regulation of the mood and the moderation of the appetite and since the serotonin is also deficient in people with depression, he must believe to a link between depression, obesity and poor nutrition.

A long time ago, animal fat would have contributed to the development of the brain of the prehistoric men; at least that is what scientists believe. Today, because of the pollution, it contributes to destroy it. Trans fat present in 40 per cent of our food products will damage the brain cells and destroy the memory.

An excess of animal fat can lead to arthritis, autoimmune diseases, psoriasis and eczema. There is no death as a result of cardiovascular diseases among the Inuit, because they eat a lot of fish.

The taking of Oil Omega, the reduction in the sugar and of the bad cholesterol can improve the sleep. The bad fats are shrink the arteries, which decreases the blood flow, and the brain is the first to suffer. It was the cause of loss of intellectual productivity.

"A brain in health depends of nutrients put at its disposal by the power supply, but also of its capacity to receive through the network of blood."[378]

A low rate of good cholesterol brings the delays in the development. The free radicals from the pollution oxidize the cells. The hypocholestérolémie impedes the development of the brain, causes of bowel problems by a rate too low in production of bile from the liver, creates deficiencies in vitamin D necessary in the absorption of calcium, because of the difficult trade between the cells and produces a lack of fluidity of cellular membranes.

The bad cholesterol interferes with the hormones, which would explain the highest rate of autism and ADHD in boys. In addition, the bad cholesterol would cause infertility.

The development of the sexual hormones is made from the good cholesterol; without cholesterol, there is not a reproduction. There are also the problems of the adrenal glands caused by an autoimmune disease and an intolerance to gluten which can lead to problems of fertility.

The junk food

We are in the era of the rapid restoration which takes the magnitude because of our style of life. It may be noted too great a consumption of sugar, additives, preservatives, without forgetting the dyes and artificial flavors. The chemicals in the power supply also alter the brain functions including food additives. The chemicals shall take the place of natural products in our plates. Among these ingredients would be the source of the hyperactivity. It is the case of the phosphate.

The phosphate in the power supply may result in brains, insomnia, aggressiveness and hyperactivity. Remove the phosphate additives in avoiding the pre-cooked dishes can lose to a child her need to take Ritalin. Phosphates are necessary, but "too it is as not enough"; this leads to behavioral disorders. The hyperactivity to phosphates affects 5 per cent of girls and up to 20% of boys, this implies that the hormones are still there for something.

The phosphate prevented the availability of calcium that is needed in the brain; that is why the milk creates difficulties with attention and hyperactivity by its high rate of phosphate. The Magnesium protects the nervous system and is essential to its balance and its proper functioning.

The lack of magnesium and zinc influence the enzyme system. The excess phosphate is a cause of osteoporosis because it influences the metabolism of OS.

Among the sensitive subjects, intoxication to the phosphate causes a disruption of metabolism by blocking the secretion of the hormone noradrenaline from the adrenal glands, which command and adjusts the flow of nerve excitations of the brain. Where a dysregulation of the behavior which is manifested as soon the withdrawal when the child goes from breast milk to milk cow. The situation is deteriorating with the normal power to 2 or 3 years (with the contribution of fortified cereals to the soy lecithin).[379]

Overdoses of phosphate may cause difficulties of language, of sleep disorders, a lacklustre, a exaggerated susceptibility, disabilities, of adaptation, of permanent distractions, violence, of hyperactivity and emotional instability. Cow's milk contains six times more phosphate than human milk. The egg yolks and legumes in also

223

contain; that is why an intolerance to eggs, to peas or the beans might be caused by the sensitivity to phosphates. Therefore, a milk allergy can lead to an allergy to the legumes and eggs.

The power supply can therefore cause handicaps. There was an increase in behavioral and academic difficulties in school. Since the 1960s, phosphates have increased by 300 per cent in the food industry, especially during the last decade. 2 to 3 children on 10 In are sensitive. The intoxication to the phosphate creates a brain dysfunction. It is better to avoid cow's milk, eggs, soft drinks, cooked ham, the lecithins, baking powder, soybeans, the MSG that is found in large quantities in the restoration, aspartame, citric acid, stabilizers, anti-caking agents, conservation officers, additives and colorants.

The phosphate is blocking the communication between the intellectual part of the brain and the one related to emotions. "Food phosphates bind to heavy metals in the body."[380]

The decline of phosphate can decrease, or even to make disappear, obsessions, the mountings and rituals . A bad intestinal bacteria love the phosphate, which allows him to spread. This Escherichia coli in too large quantity in the intestine is detrimental to the functioning of the brain and even more if the intestine is porous.

Chapter 16

The irradiation of food

Massive sterilization of food soiled

The irradiation would be a technique of food preservation. It is to decontaminate and to slow down the ripening process. This would reduce the costs of production while extending the duration of conservation, as well as the commercial life of the product. This technique would destroy the bacteria, insects and other pests. It would also make it possible to recycle outdated products.

This process also lowers the sanitary conditions as well as the vigilance, since the people who work in the food industry would no longer need to do as much attention to avoid bacterial infections during the handling of products. It is a technique used to hide the lack of hygiene and camouflage to poor sanitary conditions. The meat dirty and contaminated with feces in the slaughterhouses would thus be cleaned and disinfected. Yuck!

The aim is that the food keeps longer and s abyss less quickly during its period of storage, which allows the transport over longer distances. The Irradiation allows you to store products throughout the year to make them accessible regardless of the season. It does not prevent just the ripening process to continue, but also the potatoes to germinate, which creates black spots and rots in the inside as if the irradiated food developed a form of cancer. This gives a misleading appearance of freshness. The foods seem well from the outside while they are brown or black in the center. In addition, consumers are paying more for these foods which appear to be more healthy as they are in reality. The appearance is more important than the quality of the content. Fruit and vegetables are already dead since irradiation kills any form of life; this is why a process of decomposition at idle speed is triggered. The quality of the food is deteriorating.

A product that has respected the sanitary conditions in a reasonable time does not need to be irradiated to destroy the local economy and the life of the small growers who are invaded by foreign products.

It is once again the paranoia around the fear of small bugs that would have triggered this phenomenon of food that is not new. The main objective is to save of the losses and the money. This are of the large bugs which should be afraid: the promoters of the radioactivity. This would be the fear of the bacterium E. coli to explain the reason for the use of nuclear waste to irradiate the food, because of the lack of place for the store in a safe manner. They would like to irradiate the dangerous bacterium E. coli in foods, while they would use in laboratories for the manufacture of GMOS. Look for the error.

Irradiation is a technique which resembles the sterilization and pasteurization. The irradiation of meat would be at the same title that chlorination of the water. It is important not to confuse the ionization with the solar rays, which are a natural ionization adapted whose minimum of ions created is necessary to life.

X-rays at any power

This nuclear industry would use the radioactivity in submitting the food to a radiation of electrons in power stations of ionization using a ball of cobalt diving in the water which absorbs the rays.

In Canada, gamma rays are produced by the cobalt which is immersed in a swimming pool of 24 feet of depth. At the time to serve, the ball of cobalt out of the water and Monte in the irradiator around which circulate food. The radiation would be tantamount to 233 million chest radiographs. "This exhibition is 50 times higher than the dose required to kill a human being."[381]

The Cobalt 60 is a toxic substance and deadly. Therefore, any form of life to the inside of the food itself is killed. The electrons are projected as quickly as the speed of light. The transfer of nuclear energy by radiation causes a warming in the food as if it went to the microwave. The material of which the cell of the food undergoes a bombardment would be similar to the one used during the genetic manipulation. The Radioactivity would also be used for the bombing of the seed in the seed production of GMOS.

Approximately 40 000 tonnes of food have been irradiated in 2003. The fresh strawberries are submitted to irradiation up to 8 minutes and the frozen chicken would take 20 minutes. Most of the rice from China would have been treated as well. It is permitted to irradiate bags of earth and the pots used for culture, even sanitary products and bodily hygiene. If radioactive particles remain in the cotton of buffers, it is not surprising to note the number of cancers of the uterus and the ovaries, as well as the rate of female infertility. "The Canada authorizes the irradiation of onions, potatoes and flour."[382]

Abracadabra!

It would disappear from the food everything that there is good in him to do there appear of toxic substances. The cells of the fruit and vegetables would lose their ability to fight infections, which would promote a bacterial mutation harmful. The color, texture and taste of the food would be altered. Have you not noticed that some fruits seem to have lost their taste of origin?

At doses higher than 6 kilograms, irradiation can destroy the vitamins and other nutrients, thus decreasing the nutritional qualities of the product, without that the average consumer to be aware of it. This can then also have a negative impact on the taste, smell and texture of processed foods. For example, in France, the dose of 10 kilograms is authorized for the treatment of cereals, rice flour or spices, and the dose of 5 kilograms is authorized to deal with the meat and fish. Foods are irradiated long enough for bacteria and molds may be dead. The food is also death. For example, the Potato do more germ and the germ is necrosis in a black pulp.[383]

In the sterilization of foods, this are not just the micro-organisms which are destroyed, but also all of their nutritional values. The irradiation would eliminate the antioxidants, would transform the essential fats in the degrading treatment and would alter the structure of proteins. These are the empty calories of all nutrient values. The Irradiation has destroyed the life. We eat food which are biologically dead; this would be the same thing as biting in the carton. In addition, it gives a bitter taste to foods contributing to the whims of food. When we eat raw vegetables, it is in reality of canned, and we know that the food preserved are devitalized.

The Irradiation destroys some useful bacteria which would have allowed us to trace such food as unfit for human consumption. Fruits and vegetables are not more freshly picked and they are no longer part of a living power supply. The food is completely denatured of its biological structure deep. Why do undergo a ill-treatment to our food if essential to the maintenance of the life? "The irradiation does not merely to exterminate the unwanted germs, by the same occasion, they destroy instantly and totally vitamins, antioxidants, enzymes, fatty acids, and in the case of red meat, some components naturally present in the fibers."[384]

The lipids resent the irradiation, which also affects the carbohydrates and destroyed some of the amino acids. Irradiated foods and genetically modified organisms would be, on the plan nutritious, less good compared to food not altered, because the irradiation would produce and would alter the chemical compounds to the inside of the food.

The loss in essential nutrients is not of the irradiated food an ideal to feed the populations who are already suffering from malnutrition. Nutrient losses increase during transportation and storage. Even the smell is amended and camouflaged by other chemicals having the property to be potentially toxic.

As well, the manner in which the industry wants to use the irradiation to help the populations deficient on the nutritional plan will lead to provide them with food taurine deficient. In addition to this, the people in malnutrition have a resistance to toxins less large and therefore the irradiated foods with their radiolytic products may prove to be fatal.[385]

The ions form of the molecules that did not exist before. It would offer our assistance to these countries with food poisoned.

Vitamins are essential to our body and to its development, as well as for the maintenance of life as such. Most of the vitamins of the B complex are destroyed or, more precisely, mysteriously disappeared. It is of vitamins B1, B2, B3, B6 and B12. Almost all children with autism have a deficit of the vitamin B complex, several of which must take supplements. "Vitamins help to release the energy from our food supply and contribute to the growth, to the healing and healing. A deficiency of vitamins can lead to a health more fragile, to the weakening, to a greater susceptibility to the disease, and may ultimately lead to the death (the extreme case)."[386]

In fact, up to 80% of the vitamin A would be destroyed by the ionization, as well as 48% of the Beta Carotene: two very important elements for the development of the view. The Vitamins more rare as the K and the PP, same that the folic acid necessary for the operation of the metabolism, would also be destroyed or greatly diminished. There is a significant loss of vitamins, up to 91% for vitamin E, 90% for vitamin C (an antioxidant essential) and 95% for vitamin B1.

Vitamin C is an antioxidant indispensable in the fight against free radicals often produced inside the irradiated foods. The techniques of the food industry can impoverish the food while making it toxic. The separated molecules can unite to other with which they would normally be incompatible, leaving room for the formation of toxic chemical substances. The Irradiation degrades the quality to increase the quantity and longevity. This would therefore be a contributing factor to the nutritional deficiencies.

The enzymes contributing to their prédigestion are also destroyed or partially or completely, which can promote the triggering of allergies or intolerances. A researcher in food science has stated to me, seeing the results of the analysis of my daughter, that she would have developed allergies to all foods that are irradiated. Even the natural sugars and essential fatty acids disappear as by disenchantment. "According to the Collective against food irradiation, this irradiation destroys and alters the vitamins, proteins, essential fatty acids and other food components. But this technique can also change the taste, odour and consistency of the food in the making sometimes little appetizing."[387]

There are a lot more disadvantages than advantages to the ionization of food. It attacks the structure of cells and the breaking of the chromosomes. We do not know the profound changes in the cells of the food. The irradiation could be a poison to delay.

Of the chemistry to the menu

A radiation produced ionization in the food that he cross member. Irradiation can produce ions, uproot the neutrons and change the DNA in cells causing cuts in those, which may cause mutations by recombination between the bacteria that are resistant to it. "Finally, the ionization could disrupt the genetic heritage of bacteria and fungi; the latter can mutate, creating a risk of new diseases."[388]

The judgment of the multiplication of certain cells to rapid division introduced foreign elements. The break in the molecules can form of free radicals. This disturbance in the molecules can therefore create toxic substances. The chromosomes of cells break and this would be risky if it occurs a mutation of new viruses or bacteria. It will be possible to establish a link with new viruses and bacteria, or even the creation of new diseases. The risks are still unknown and due to a serious change in their composition which would appear of compounds that can cause of genetic disorders, which has been observed in laboratory rats. "A particular substance created by the irradiation in food, the alkylcyclobutane, could be a factor of cancer."[389]

Damage to cells and genes would be caused by the free radicals produced in foods as a result of the irradiation. The irradiation would have a cytotoxic effect and génétoxique. Their consumption could result in genetic damage in the cells of the men. The exposures to high doses of energy can cause the formation of unique radiolytic products and not existing in a natural way in the food. One of these specific products to irradiated foods promotes the development of cancers and genetic damage in rats. Damage cellular and genetic can also occur in humans.

A peroxide oxidizing the cellular components the more sensitive would also be created inside the irradiated food, from cells of microorganisms. The other toxic products that can be found inside the irradiated foods would be the peroxide, the cyclobutanome, toluene and the méthylkétane, all suspected in the problems of birth and those related to the formation of cancers.

"The irradiation also causes some volatile agents which may be toxic, according to the type of packaging. There may be formation of benzene, formaldehyde, octane, butane and Methyl propane in some foods."[390]

Ionizing radiation can uproot the electrons of the atoms in the material crossing. They destroy the matter first to create chemical compounds new. The pieces of molecules become of the electrons and the free radicals. They are very reactive and can recombine and become toxic. Free radicals in reaction with food can create new chemical substances. The benzene, which would be present in the beef irradiated, is a substance known for its carcinogenic properties. Liver cancer is caused by the aflatoxins which are often produced by food irradiation, which also transforms the nitrates to nitrites which have the function to be mutagenic. They react with amino acids and proteins to transform itself into a carcinogenic substance, the nitrosamine. In the process of turning cancerous, this are the lesions are created which may lead to the death of the cell or cause its mutation. Free radicals create genetic alterations that can cause cell damage and damage to the DNA. "The irradiation of food is a technique which puts in motion the free radicals of foods so that they destroy all living things: enzymes, good bacteria."[391]

The being who consumes would receive these free radicals. This is not just the DNA of the food which is disturbed, but also the one who is feeding. Any food whose DNA has been disrupted can change the human genome. We are what we eat and we therefore to become beings mutants. "Mutations exist in nature; subject to a climate stress for example, plants adapt their genome, mutate or express other genes that were in sleep."[392]

But, unfortunately, by the genetic disruption, the plant and the animal lose their faculties of adaptation. The pathogens can be develop, because their enemies have been dislodged, since the good bacteria are also destroyed. The imbalance between the good and bad bacteria makes the food more vulnerable to contamination during the manipulation, because the food has lost its natural defenses. Any living being houses an ecosystem that we must not interfere. This are not all of the microorganisms contained in the food that are harmful, because some have useful features and this are the strongest and most ill who resist. It is still a technique which destroys the life of non-target organisms. This process could also create strains of mutant bacteria even more difficult to destroy against which the body would be possibly without resources.

"Some insects may not respond as expected and modify their defense, for example, by immunizing, in producing more of poison or making it much more destructive."[393]

These foods and their toxic compounds could therefore cause damage to our organs and systems. Nuclear power is used in the treatment of cancers while he destroyed both the healthy cells that cancer cells, causing recurrences very profitable for the industry. The Treatment The most popular against cancer would cause cancer. Beautiful aberration!

Smile, you are X-ray

Any irradiation can cause cancer, leukaemia and malformations on the genetic plan.

Scientific tests carried out in the course of the last thirty years have demonstrated that the absorption of irradiated foods caused a myriad of problems: a higher rating of genetic mutations and dysfunctions of the reproductive system in rats, a high level of embryonic death in mice and a chromosomal aberration affecting the human blood cells. It has also been proven that irradiation destroys vitamins and creates sub-products, such as the cyclobutanones which are linked to cancer of the colon.[394]

Irradiation is also used to disinfect the cereals such as wheat. Irradiated foods may change the composition of blood.

At the end of four weeks, blood samples were collected and four of the five children who ate of the irradiated wheat have presented a large chromosomal polyploidy, as well as other abnormal cells. Once the irradiated wheat removed from their power, it took 24 weeks before that the blood of children by having consumed returns to normal and that all the abnormal cells have completely disappeared.[395]

If the wheat is not genetically modified, it is when the same by irradiation. The training of new molecules has created 65 volatile substances that have been found in irradiated foods by the American army. The volatile substances would be more toxic than those who are not.

Radioactive particles are metabolized by our Organization as if it were of minerals. The food can be contaminated by radioactivity or by what it does produce in them. The molecules are looking for partners to recombine and create items new biochemical. Of molecules newly created can attach themselves on the thyroid and the damage by taking the place of the iodine. Radioactive iodine can take the place of the potassium iodine in the thyroid gland, which would explain the high rate of cancer of the thyroid gland. The Good iodine supports the body against the microbial attacks, parasitic and viral diseases. The iodine can be deficient in several children with autism. Thus, the radiation changes the iodine from the thyroid, whereas the iodine has as a function to protect the gland against the irradiation. Another molecule would take the place of the calcium in our OS that can make them cancerous. A radioactive molecule has a chemical property which resembles that of calcium and which may be considered by our Organization that it thwarts as such. It is dangerous to irradiate fungi because they are true sponges that can absorb the radioactivity. And yet, they make us believe that the food contains not of radioactivity. The Berlingots of milk have been recalled because they were contaminated by radiation.

"However, the ionizing radiation High-energy can lead to the creation of radioactivity in the matter bombed. If the radioactive source was damaged, the food could be contaminated by radioactivity."[396]

The industry of the disease

The following problems have been observed in animals consuming irradiated food: a degradation of the immune system, growth disorders, a dietary deficiency and a degradation of the genetic makeup of the cells that lead to aberrations in the chromosomes that could lead to an incompatibility of reproduction, therefore a infertility.

"Laboratory Animals fed irradiated food on long periods of time suffer from genetic diseases, problems of reproduction, deformations and early mortality."[397] Of mice fed the irradiated wheat have had more of mortality in the progeny and have developed tumors. The hens fed irradiated wheat have lost more of embryos. The effects are both mutagenic and toxic. A change in the size of the ovaries was noticed in rodents fed with irradiated potatoes.

The Cobalt 60 may produce inflammations to the tissues of the brain. The Irradiation, disrupting the functioning of living cells, modifies the chemical functions. The content of new substances can lead to mutations and cancers. The cell wall being damaged, its repair is sometimes partial and only becomes a cancerous that several years later. The cell membrane damaged makes the kernel vulnerable to attacks of free radicals. The immune system no longer knows to face the mortalities Cellular, because they are too numerous. When the cell is stressed, its mechanisms of adaptation and defense are overloaded with work and therefore to the limits of their abilities. The body no longer knows face the aggressors that it no longer recognizes. The exposure to even small doses, who end up also by accumulate in the tissues, makes our system more susceptible to infections. Sterilize the food may therefore cause risks to health. "The developing fetus are especially radiosensitive,; the risks linked to are the miscarriage, mental retardation, malformations, a delay of growth."[398]

The peroxidase which is done inside the irradiated foods and fixed ingested an excessive amount of oxygen making it inaccessible to the cells of the body and can cause of psychiatric disorders by premature aging of cells. It would be one of the causes of the Depression. The peroxidase escapes the enzymes and antioxidants become absent of food by irradiation itself, which is not the case when the peroxidation is natural instead of be created artificially. The quality of the communication between cells is diminished.

The Cells speak between them without stops according to a molecular language whose accuracy allows you to maintain the balance within the organization. The release of these interactions between cells seems to be linked to the accumulation of free radicals eager to oxygen in the cellular membranes which blurs the communications, disrupts the interactions between cells and the mechanisms repairers to accident and, thus, accelerates the aging of the affected tissue. The ionizing radiation, when it reaches the members of brain cells, cause irreversible damage.[399]

Irradiation kills the cell to its mode of division; she can create muscular atrophies, affect the nervous systems and gastro-intestinal tract and cause lung disorders. The changes or disturbances can genetic be transmitted from one generation to the other, but there is less chance when the infertility affects 60% to 100% of persons exposed to irradiation.

Free radicals cause damage and alter the cell membrane of the DNA and detrimental to the synthesis of the enzymes and proteins. Antioxidants help the production of enzymes that are too often destroyed by free radicals themselves. The Vitamins removed from food by the ionization would have helped in the fight against the oxidation, which has been caused by irradiation. During the last 50 years, dozens of experiments have been conducted on animals fed with irradiated food to demonstrate that the irradiation would involve risks for the health. Among these disorders, were identified damage to organs, tumors, disorders of the immune system, reproductive problems, genetic mutations and premature death.

Cats fed with irradiated meat have suffered neurological disorders. One thing is for sure is that the Australian cats, them, does not seem to really not appreciate of irradiated foods. In the country of kangaroos, irradiation of food for animals has long been mandatory, until the time when the company has withdrawn from the market its products intended for cats in November 2008. The reason? An investigation of the grouping of Australian veterinary had found of neurological disorders on cats fed with irradiated foods at high doses by this firm.[400]

Here is the assessment of the consequences in Australia on cats fed with the irradiated meat: 90 cats have been seriously sick whose 30 have been forced to be euthanized. The diseases observed are a loss of muscle coordination, paralysis of the lower limbs and four members, loss of the use of the view; these symptoms would not be emerged that four months later.

Nothing is 100% SAFE

If it uses nuclear weapons is that the destroyed nuclear life. "There are many projects to use the irradiation in other areas, such as the soil sterilization to eliminate weed seeds, insects and fungi."[401]

The seeds of irradiated foods may not germinate; this will be the destruction of natural environments and the disruption of ecosystems. Also, the transportation of nuclear material is potentially dangerous for the environment, because it can be at the origin of an ecological disaster is serious and irreparable. After a few months, the radioactive substance must be replaced as well as the water in which it has been retained. What do they do with this substance? The discharge-they in the course of the water after the allegedly well filtered?

It seems that, in some countries, those who practice the irradiation of foods are treated as criminals. Why is it not as well among us? What happens the day where farmers will to irradiate their fields with nuclear substances to come to the end of diseases, insects and parasites of their crops on which pesticides no longer have the effect? There are fears about the long term negative consequences on health and with respect to the loss of nutrient values.

In Canada, the ground beef, poultry, flours, shrimp and prawns and mangoes would be the foods most irradiated. Be used to camouflage the dirty conditions of some of the factories and some slaughterhouses.

We must wait 20 years before to see the harmful effects on health. 20 to 50 million deaths would have been caused by the pharmaceutical industry, which represents much more damage that could cause a virus on the planetary plane.

The WHO would refuse always to consider the private studies and non-subsidized by the industry in question which issue warnings and approve when even this technique.

How the irradiated foods have they been able to be declared healthy and safe, while the tests carried out already in the 1950s showed that the animals consuming irradiated foods were suffering of tens of health problems, including premature deaths, mutations or other genetic abnormalities, of the dead fetuses, and other reproductive problems, problems of immune system, internal bleeding death, of organic depredations, tumors, of the problems of growth and nutritional deficiencies?[402]

The Who would have also declined the arms before the pressure of the nuclear industries in abandoning a research program in 1961 concerning the toxicity, the problems of genetic mutations and nutrient deficiencies of irradiated foods in order to permit this practice. After the scandals surrounding the H1N1, it is very difficult to repeat confidence in Health Canada and to the World Health Organization. Although the safety of food as well processed has never been proven, scientists tell us: "Trust us!" throughout my life, I have learned to be wary of people who tell me that. The dose of acceptable radiation would only concern the economic interests.

The irradiation of food would serve more to sponsors and manufacturers of cobalt 60, and C is the disinformation of the public which would create the greater margin of profits. "The uncertainty as to the Security never appear in the reports of international organizations advocating the irradiation."[403]

The irradiation involves risks in the short, medium and long terms on the environment and for the health of the citizens and the workers who are in contact with these hazardous products. The workers of nuclear plants could reduce the radiation at home and in their vehicle.

Tests on the immediate toxicity would have been made on irradiated food while it is practically impossible since an irradiated food may not be eaten two weeks after its treatment because of the rate too high in toxins and free radicals. How have they done to measure the toxicity of these products in the short term? No study would have been made concerning their harmful effects in the long term because it is impossible to predict the biochemical reaction in the long term to the interior of a body as a result of the Radioactive treatments.

More than 90 per cent of food borne illnesses - and therefore the food-borne diseases in the sense defined by the World Health Organization - have as a point of origin to the House and the restoration. This means that a food, that it has been irradiated or not, if the handling in a restaurant or at home is erroneous, will not change strictly nothing, regardless of whether it has been irradiated or not.[404]

Organic agriculture could not even prove that it does not use this technique. Spices would be fumigated with the oxide of methylene although this practice is prohibited in the United States. It would not be allowed to radiate of organic foods while farmers would not have to be able on the packaging and storage techniques. To be sure, it should avoid the fruit out of season as the exotic fruits and the fruits of the fields in full winter, including those from other countries. Foods derived from livestock and organic agriculture would contain 87% more vitamins, minerals and essential fat that the other products, including more of iron and calcium.

235

It would not have been possible to prove the safety of plastic packages that cover the foods during treatments by ionization. Is it that the toxic materials of packaging can penetrate the food? "However, the irradiation process requires in reality the use of food additives Extra to check the adverse effects."[405]

The foods are less nutritious and there is fighting for the transport to the other end of the world. The transport of these materials radio-active in boats or trains would represent a factor of risk of accidents and potential attacks. The pollution as a result of a nuclear accident and the transport of cobalt will be irreparable. The radioactive fallout would be more important when a transportation accident that this was the case for the Chernobyl accident. Thousands of hectares of soils are likely to be contaminated.

"These accidents causing great concern on the impact radio-active possible on soils of North Americans and Europeans (in case of rain) which discharge toxic components contained in the radioactive clouds from the Japan."[406]

The transport of hazardous materials represents the risks to health and the environment since it also contributes greatly to the pollution and global warming. The transport of radioactive materials is not without serious risks. The soil, the water and the air can become contaminated. A rich soil retains more pollutants. Radioactive atoms present in the soil can be absorbed by the plant.

The plants of irradiation can be a factor of air pollution and environmental. The nuclear industry product of the tons of radioactive waste. The nuclear would reject of the CO2 that night to the ozone layer. China has 60 plants of irradiation. A certain quantity of radioactivity may be rejected in the air and the water course.

The radioactive food rejected eventually ended up in the food chain. The Uranium Mines leach their wastewater in the rivers in Tibet, of people are pumped. The dead water would become black, such as spots inside the irradiated potatoes. Animals and plants would be dead suddenly of unknown cause. "The radioactive waste dumped at random near water courses pollute rivers, lakes and sources."[407]

It takes tens of millions of years before that the radioactivity disappears from the environment. The radioactive waste are not recyclable. Researchers would not even have found reliable ways to bury them. For storage, the concrete containers are leakproof as for 10 years and those in metal can rust quickly. The Landfill in depth is not guaranteed, because the sealing of containers may change under the ground, as well as the stability of the ground, and we do not know the interactions with the different chemical elements sub-land.

"Radioactivity will recover inevitably to the surface in a contaminant of uncontrollable way the vital elements (water, soil, etc.) on very large territories."[408]

The nuclear installations are dangerous: their security is insufficient and the risks are really badly calculated. This are the most hazardous materials that man has created and this are our children who will have to live with this situation.

Chapter 17

The Microwave Oven

The chemical transformation of food

Methods of culinary preparations may have adverse effects on the food. The dishes are cooked or heated by friction between the cells, because that is what creates the heat. The broken molecules would escape the vitamins. Cooking by microwave would therefore contribute to a loss of nutrient values. If the molecular structure is torn or transformed, our system will not be able to recognize it. By this very fact, the digestion and assimilation of food would be made difficult. The atoms as well separated can unite to other with which they are incompatible thus creating a chemical substance that can be toxic. So that is another possible form of food poisoning.

It is our current way of life that pushes us as well to save time in the preparation of our food. It is used a lot in the restoration to win precisely the time and energy. Despite the conflicting opinions between scientific researchers and the proponents of the industry from the microwave oven, Russia is one of the countries to have completely banned its use in 1976. Those who have discovered his misdeeds would have been threatened by the manufacturers. The industry of the microwave represents billions of dollars.

The cells, the atoms and molecules are irradiated by an electromagnetic radiation. The molecules in the food are shake by a vibration that would force the cells to change the polarity of the billions of times each second. It is the friction between the molecules that creates the heat. The Friction break the molecules important. The oscillation can tear and deform the molecular structures of food. The change space in the protein would become the same as that of prions leading to the production of free radicals. This cooking technique therefore would alter the chemistry of food. The radiolytic products are the new compounds formed by this mutation unknown which is not present in nature. This would be the same process, or a similar used in the genetic modification, which breaks the cells to neutralize their source of life in order to be better able to manipulate their genome. The food which fate of this oven would have suffered a change.

Who wins loses

Since the cooking is not uniform, Cold areas are created inside, which is subject to the microbial blooms. Food should not be heated more than two times to avoid microbial proliferation which multiplies each warming.

In addition, foods which have spent by the Microwave have changed of taste and they would retain less long in the refrigerator, because they would have lost their means of natural defense. It is as if a process of accelerated decomposition was initiated, similar to that which happens to the result of the irradiation of food. Microwave cooking would promote an increase of parasites, yeasts, molds, bacteria and viruses, because their enemies who would normally have fought have been destroyed and thus eliminated whose beneficial bacteria to our intestinal flora. This cooking not uniform would contribute to food poisoning.

The plastic would be extremely toxic especially if it is heated. How many dishes are heated in the microwave ovens even their containing plastic? Many parents have done heat the breast milk, preparations for infant and cow's milk in bags or bottles in plastic with the microwave oven. In addition to intoxicate their baby, the vitamins and the immune transfer of the mother to the child would thus have been destroyed, without speaking of molecular changes making these Milks If difficult to digest. The components of the plastic containers may migrate into the food as well heated. "Several chemical components are used for the manufacture of plastic materials, and some of them can cause cancer. It is not impossible that these chemicals are able to go to the outside of the container and seep into the foods that are there."[409]

The food can therefore absorb the quantities of chemical substances in the plastic during the firings. Warm up of breast milk in the microwave can cause damage in its molecular structure during and even after the heating. "Microwave ovens are not recommended to heat the bottle of a baby. [...] Can cause slight changes in the milk. In the formulas for infants, there may be a loss of some vitamins. In the breast milk, some properties immunity can be destroyed."[410]

This may therefore destroy the capacity of the Child to combat the diseases. "Another study in Vienna has demonstrated that heat of breast milk in the microwave can lead to changes structured, functional and immunity and that the transform microprobes amino acids L-proline in D-proline, a toxin attacker the nervous system, the liver and the kidneys."[411]

The alterations of proteins and peptides can represent certain dangers Since the D-proline is a neurotoxin. More in-depth studies should take place regarding these molecular alterations that would affect also other compounds such as amino acids. Concerning the soybeans, the protein would be denatured, as for the milk, and could become toxic to the kidneys and the liver and dangerous on the plan of the Immunity (cancer, leukemia...).

The losses in vitamins are numerous. High temperatures and intense do not alter only the structures of proteins, but also would destroy the vitamins, especially vitamin C, and also the B1, B6 and B12, deficient in autistic children. A decrease of 20 per cent of the vitamin B2 and the destruction of folic acid have been found in the milk for infants. The Microwave Oven would thus represent another form of nutrient deficit. It would destroy also with components of melatonin if necessary to sleep.

"Two researchers, White and Hertel, have confirmed that the cooking in a microwave oven significantly changes the substance of nutritious food."[412] The live food become dead and denatured. The worst enemy of vitamins is the intense heat which can destroy up to 95 per cent of vitamins B1 and C. Food, which have undergone a profound change, are devitalized. Those who say that microwave cooking does not create a nutrient deficit contradict themselves by saying that the intensive heat destroyed almost all the vitamins. Any form of cooking may distort the molecules of the food. "A loss of 97% of Antioxidants (flavonoids) of broccoli has been observed with a cooking in the micro-waves against 66% with cooking in boiling water."[413]

There is therefore a loss between 60% and 90% of the vital energy of a food product, which would represent a destruction of micronutrients. This method of cooking also destroyed the digestive enzymes in addition to destroy the essential proteins to the growth of the baby. Certain foods cooked or heated as well would become indigestible. If our organization is unable to assimilate the denatured foods is that he would consider as aggressors which grow to produce of leukocytes that can trigger food allergies. People have developed a sensitivity to food passed to the micro-waves whose signs of allergies ranging up to 99% of persons tested.

The food would become foreigners and unknown by our digestive system because of the profound alteration of their chemical composition. A decline in the general state of health would have appeared among people who often use this oven. We would have noted among they a weakening of the immune system, a food poisoning, degeneration of the nervous system, cases of cancer, chronic fatigue as well as a transformation of blood cells. This technology would be one of the most important causes of poor health.

It would affect the flow of calcium in the cells and would reduce the level of hemoglobin.

The red blood cells are corrupted and their number decreases by the radiation exposure of the microwave. And they are the ones who are responsible for the transport of oxygen to the brain as well as to other bodies, which can produce a mental fog, the inability to concentrate, vertigo, nausea, as many symptoms found in chronic fatigue syndrome.[414]

The Microwave Would form more radilite as the other modes of cooking. This can cause a deterioration of the immune system as well as of the anemia. In addition, it diminishes the capacity of the body to use vitamins and minerals.

It emanates from the microwave frequencies close to those of mobile phones also incriminated in the development of tumors of the brain. This would be of irradiated foods that irradieraient also their tower; it would therefore be of a direct form of irradiation, the consequences of which are always ignored or not admitted. "No cell of a living organism would not be able to withstand the destructive forces of such a power."[415]

The devices are not waterproof to 100%. It can therefore absorb this energy which is negative at doses significant.

"As in the case of foods, this energy is transformed into heat in the blood. The sensitive parts of the body, for example, the eyes, the testes and the brain, are not able to eliminate the additional heat that can accumulate."[416]

In the vicinity of a microwave oven, the operation of a pacemaker can be disrupted and thus send false sequences in the heart. The devices are not waterproof to 100%. Of Drugs or supplements placed near the oven can lose their effectiveness. Once connected, the kiln may issue an electromagnetic field in a circumference of up to 5 meters.

The Digestive disorders may be such that a formation of cancer of the stomach or intestines can ensue. The Digestive disorders are often expressed by a feeling of heaviness in the stomach and a long digestion. The enzymes of digestion of food are destroyed, but also those products in us by the consumption of these foods. We should not eat a food to the inside of several minutes after its output of the oven, therefore when it begins to cool, because the microwave would remain active and could continue to cook everything they touch on their passage, therefore to change the structure of our cells. Fats would suffer a duplication thus creating substances cancerous.

All types of waves can be dangerous: it depends on the intensity and duration of the exposure. The leakage of a few watts are possible from the walls of the device or a door improperly watertight or by the use of an old device. "The metal mesh in front of the screen do not prevent the leaks perfectly. So, the more we get away from the oven, the more we ensures to be the less exposed as possible to the leaks, since these decrease with distance."[417]

Our organs capture the airwaves. Before an open door of a microwave that cannot operate if the door is not closed, a rat placed at 50 cm would be death of generalized hyperthermia.

Repeated abortions can occur in women which this type of oven is placed at the same level as their hips. The standards concerning the leaks would be different from one country to another; that is why it is necessary to pay attention to the location where the device has been purchased.

"On 2043 children, it has been observed 33 cases of neonatal deaths or major malformations, the only fact explaining this abnormal proportion being the most frequent use of equipment to short wave in the mothers of these children."[418]

A decline in libido would also have been noticed as well as lesions in the Genital cells. Here is the list of all the causes that would be related to the use of this method of cooking in the long term: increase the bad cholesterol to the detriment of a decrease in the good cholesterol, eye fatigue, affection of the central nervous system, change in blood chemistry, damage to cells, weakening of the immune system, degenerative diseases and malfunctions in the lymphatic system, development of cancer cells, weight gain, behavioral disorders, insomnia, brain lesions that can lead to seizures, disturbances of growth hormones, increase in white blood cells as if they were responding to a infection. It may also attack the spleen According to Doctors of Traditional Chinese Medicine.

241

Of the seeds that have dipped in the water that has spent in the microwave, although cooled, have not germinated compared to those soaked in water from the tap. Then, imagine the damage that this can do to your body.

Conclusion

The autism would be a disease invented, or rather created by man, by his recklessness and by its indifference. It is high time that we realize of all the evil that was done. Our children we send signs; still it is necessary to listen and see to understand. Autism is a chemical intoxication, food and environmental. It is a physical disease of modern times which has an impact on the development and operation of the brain.

When Albert Einstein predicted that the human being was going to destroy itself, he thought to autoimmune diseases where our body produces antibodies against its own cells? Is this that autism would be the beginning of the end? In order to survive, the planet will have to find a way to get rid of us if we do not change in time. To do this, it would have found, for the moment, the cancer and infertility. Me, I believe that it is the money which destroys the world now. And you?

To force to let us do so without saying anything, without action, we are all responsible for autism. We will feel finally free the day where we will cease to be afraid.

* * *

www.ingramcontent.com/pod-product-compliance
Lightning Source LLC
Chambersburg PA
CBHW060830170526
45158CB00001B/127